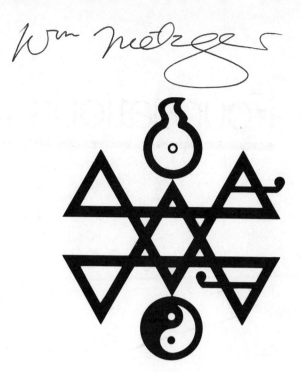

Foundations for Holistic

Health Nursing Practices

The Renaissance Nurse

Dolores Krieger

Ph.D., R.N.
Professor of Nursing
Department of Research and Theory Development in Nursing Science
Division of Nursing
New York University
New York City

With clinical papers
by seven holistic health nurses

J. B. Lippincott Company
Philadelphia   Toronto

To Martha E. Rogers, D.Sc., R.N.
pioneer nurse for a new age

6 5 4 3 2

Library of Congress Cataloging in Publication Data

Krieger, Dolores.
    Foundations for holistic health nursing practices.

    Includes index.
    1. Nursing—Philosophy.   2. Holistic medicine.
I. Title.   [DNLM: 1. Holistic health—Nursing texts.
2. Philosophy, Nursing. WY 86 K92f]
RT84.5.K74   610.73′01   81–456
ISBN 0-397-54341-7   AACRI

Printed in the United States of America

Contents

Contributors of Clinical Papers, Part 3

Nancy E. Boyd, M.A., R.N.
Instructor, Division of Nursing, New York University, New York City

Lynn Wilson Brallier, M.S.N., R.N.
Director, Stress Management Center of Metropolitan Washington; Independent Practitioner in Psychotherapy and Biofeedback, Washington, D.C.

Cathleen A. Fanslow, M.A., R.N.
Clinical Nursing Specialist and Nurse Counselor in private practice, Oncology-Thanatology, Glen Oaks, New York

Patricia Heidt, Ph.D., R.N.
Private Practitioner in Psychotherapy, New York City

Janet A. Macrae, M.A., R.N.
Practitioner and Teacher of Therapeutic Touch, fulltime Doctoral Candidate at New York University, New York City

Catherine Salveson, M.S., R.N.
Director, Senior Day Care Programs, Albuquerque-Bernalillo County Office of Senior Affairs, Albuquerque, New Mexico

Janet F. Quinn, M.A., R.N.
Instructor, Hunter College-Bellevue School of Nursing; Private Practitioner and Lecturer on Therapeutic Touch, New York City

Preface

The application of holistic philosophy to health care is not new. It is as old as the history of thinking humanity.

Human beings have always found meaning in their personal interactions (their oneness) with the universe. The exception to this is found within the rigid, dualistic world view of cartesian philosophy. Put forth and pursued by Descartes 400 years ago, the cartesian philosophy and a mechanistic view of the world have been routinely accepted in the Western world until recently. That this cartesian view of a dichotomy of mind and body is not appropriate to the study of human beings can be inferred from the increasing reluctance of contemporary scientists to continue in that mold. The rate of disavowal of this dualism seems to be proportionate to the growing recognition that any comprehensive discourse on human beings is made in reference to matter, energy, and consciousness as they relate to time and space.

The frame of reference of reality in people's everyday lives is molded by the perspective of time. In the world of linear sequence, time is defined by the drip-drip-drip of water or the mechanistic rhythm of the tick-tock of a clock. Within this structure, cause and effect can be cloaked by simplistic logic. However, if the context is that of an open, living system according to which the individual is an organization of subsystems and energies in ceaseless motion, the reference frame must be the process in its entirety, the "whole person." This, then, allows for variants at each moment of time, and, furthermore, the significance of simultaneous life events (coincidences) lies in the meanings that involved individuals assign to them.

Since the basis for the development of theory in nursing is the study of humans in their full complexity, it is to the healing of this whole person that I direct this book. The perspective of this book is a holistic one that discusses human embryologic development in Chapter 1 and then follows the life continuum through to death in Chapter 17. It sweeps the spectrum of human time from the prehistoric to the present in order to propose the foundations for modern holistic health nursing.

A background of the holistic health approach as it began in primitive cultures and as it developed in the Far East and the Mediterranean area is presented in Part 1. Shamanism, the most primitive of holistic health practices, is discussed both as it was first practiced and as it continues to be practiced in present-day cultures such as among the Amerindians. The macrocosm-microcosm paradigm and the theories behind *yin-yang* are representative of the Chinese influence, and yoga and the universal law of karma are among the ideas suggested by the Indian sphere of influence. The Egyptian and Greek spectra of holism are referred to, as well as the Renaissance with its cartesian influence and the subsequent decline of holism. Although the various civilizations presented in Part 1 were distant from each other, their concepts were similar and overlapped in many instances.

Part 2 advances the holistic framework as it is developing in contemporary society. The major avenues and many other current modalities of holistic health practice are put forward. The relationship of the Rogerian conceptual system to holistic nursing is discussed. The ancient concept of the universal order of the world and the modern consensus of open systems tending toward order are integrated in the various modalities practiced by holistic health nurses. Thus, Part 2 ends with a discussion of "what" and "who" the Renaissance Nurse is.

In Part 3, the interactions of holistic health are demonstrated in clinical papers on the holistic health nursing perspective. The chapters in Part 3 have been written by seven nurses who practice and teach in various fields of holistic health. The sampling covers Therapeutic Touch, imagery, stress management theories, the holistic conceptual framework as it is utilized in the four phases of the nursing process, the application of holism in a neighborhood setting, interaction with the elderly, and holistic methods to be used with the dying.

The crux of the holistic experience lies in its transformative elements. As holistic nurses grow in their own "wholeness," they find their perceptions and skills in the art of healing expanding. Therefore, it seems appropriate that Renaissance Nurses of this modern age should revitalize the humanism of nursing with the philosophy of holism. This holistic approach can be applied through nursing plans, research proposals, or teaching outlines.

Nursing in the holistic framework is a unique opportunity to serve, and it is an exciting challenge. There is a growing number of Renaissance Nurses today. I hope that the readers of this book will be prompted to join the ranks.

Dolores Krieger, Ph.D., R.N.

Part 1
Background of the Holistic Health Perspective

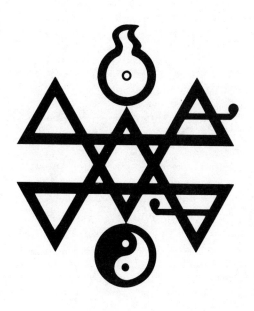

1 Introduction to the Holistic Approach

There is always an air of excitement and anticipation as revolutionary ways of thinking are translated into common language. Common folk begin to feel the impact of the new perspective in their daily lives, experience the new modeling, and therefore know it to be so. Such in fact is the state of affairs today relative to the concept of holism that underlies the idea of holistic health practices.

Strangely, the message is not new. It is as old as the history of man's thinking; however, with the rise of modern science in the sixteenth century, it was pushed aside in the Western world in favor of a more mechanistic and therefore partial view. The sixteenth century was a time of "contemplation of brute fact," as Whitehead puts it, and its thrust "was based on a recoil from the inflexible rationalization of medieval thought." This revolt was anti-rationalist, even anti-intellectual in nature. Although one result of this reaction was the birthing of modern science, it is nevertheless true that ". . . science thereby inherited the bias of thought to which it owes its origin."[1]

The men of that new age pursued isolated facts with a fervor. This willingness to delimit scientific search to objective physicochemical realities (*i.e.,* whatever one could validate by one's senses) bore fruit in the rapid growth of the industrial age and a concomitant relative economic uplift for all classes of people. Because this scientific materialism worked, until quite recent times its laws were felt to be inviolable and were applied to all manner of human concerns.

The dramatic advances in technology that characterize the twentieth century have given us a new vista of the universe and have enabled us to conceive beyond the level of mere organized common sense. Sophisticated instrument design has helped us to envision and deal with micro- as well as macro-universes. However, as scientists now delve in depth into previously unexplored and unquestioned territories of research, their findings throw a veil of doubt over traditional materialistic methods of scientific inquiry. In an increasingly sharp shift we now begin to recognize that we "forgot" to include a living context for all our logical discernments. We forgot that in living nature it is the *plan of the whole* to which its subsystems relate. In other words, it is within the context of the whole system that the subsystems have meaning.

In terms of humans, the *plan of the whole* means that practices to support a person's health must keep the self-identity of the "whole" person in mind and must recognize that it is from this enduring perspective that each individual perceives intrinsic reality. This intrinsic reality, based as it is upon the individual's life history, in turn lends the individual personality a unity of character for its expression. Consequently, the emerging stance of the holistic health practitioner is to strive to understand simultaneously the relationship of the "part" of the individual under concern to the totality of that individual's interactions and the relationship of the whole to its parts. This may be a feat tantamount to an attempt to see out of both ends of a telescope at the same time, and perhaps as ridiculous. Actually, the way is more elegant if we let nature be our teacher. As we shall see in the following pages, once we are willing to give up our restrictive modes of thinking in which only one idea is tolerated at a time, we shall be closer to a natural view of phenomena, for that is the way nature herself acts; the only realities are the connectivities between isolated events and the relationships between them.[2] Holism is implicit in every facet of life.

Holism as Law

In Human Embryologic Development

Humans by nature are whole; becoming "unwhole" must be learned.

During human embryologic development, there is nothing that describes the development process more accurately than to say that it is characterized by a holism within which every factor in the system is intrinsically related to every other factor, whether that factor is latent or actualized. In actuality, at conception and shortly thereafter every cell has the potentiality for assuming the function of every other cell. It is during the second week following conception that a decisive differentiation of the cells occurs. This critical moment arrives with exact precision as the inside and the outside of the growing cluster of cells (the *endoderm* and the *ectoderm* of the embryonic disk) arrange themselves in such a way that a third germ layer, the *mesoderm,* will develop along a longitudinal demarcation called the *primitive streak.* This primitive streak becomes the precursor of the spinal cord. A remarkable transformation occurs at this time: according to precisely timed ordering principles the dynamics of which are not known in detail, a sequential differentiation of cells into specific tissues and organs occurs. The physiologic center for the intelligent control of this highly integrated development is the primitive streak. In an exquisitely programmed outreach into the space of the growing embryo, each of the three rapidly differentiating germ layers spins out specific tissues in a stunning display of closely timed coordination to lay down the living fabric of the growing organism. The warp is fit into the woof with amazing speed and accuracy, and by the eighth week of development almost all of the organs are formed and the embryo is recognizable as human.

At full term, the human baby will have grown from a single fertilized ovum to an integrated being comprised of over 6,000 billion cells whose future growth and development throughout the entire life span will continue to be characterized by an intrinsic holism.[3]

In Human Neurologic Function

The unitary nature of the growing being is graphically portrayed in its functioning as well as in its form. This can be demonstrated in the functional responses of the nervous system which always maintains a special reference to the person as a whole. All behavior is meaningfully coordinated in every moment of the individual's existence. When this is not the case, the disruption is considered to be pathologic or to indicate a severe disintegration of the system.

There is considerable cause to wonder at the constancy of this holistic frame of reference in which the human has being, because the intricate coordinate efforts that shape behavior may bring response from elements derived from very different embryonic origins. For instance, during one simple reflex act, neurons derived from the ectoderm, muscles derived from the mesoderm, and endocrine glands derived from the endoderm work in unitary fashion.

In Human Biochemical Modeling

As the cell is traced back to its molecular constituents, one is impressed by the wholeness that governs the dynamic functions, which at this level of organization are essentially those of wave phenomena. Here one's attention is caught not only by the holism that governs the human physical being but also by a unified paradigm in reference to the life process itself which transcends species.

For instance, there is a biochemical holism among all land organisms, including humans. All contain approximately twenty of the same chemical elements and, in addition, both the ratios in which these chemicals occur and the functions that they perform are similar. Analysis indicates that very few chemicals—carbon, oxygen, hydrogen, nitrogen, sulfur, and phosphorus—make up the basic molecules of all terrestrial organisms. This choice of chemical elements cannot be considered a chance event, for the tetravalent structure allowed by the four bonding sites of carbon, the electrophilic properties of hydrogen, the nucleophilic properties of oxygen and nitrogen, and the innovative structuring allowed by the covalent bond are not to be found in such equally functional form anywhere else in the entire periodic table of chemical elements.[4]

Furthermore, there is, a strong similarity in ionic exchange, the way the waveforms we call atoms interact in the body (Table 1–1). The positive ions are most often sodium, potassium, and calcium; the negative ions are made up of chlorides, carbonates, phosphates, and sulfates. Together these ions exert a chemical control on the electrical neutrality of body fluids and cells, both of which are important in the specific maintenance of liquid volume in the various body fluid systems critical to the living process. The consistency with which exclusion of other possibilities occurs in nature indicates a logically coherent modeling.

Other than the previously stated conditions, there are only about a half dozen other elements—iron, zinc, cobalt, magnesium, and other trace elements—constituting organisms. There is no known land organism in which there is an absolute nonexistence of water. Even a dry seed is said to consist of over 20% water, and the composition of the human body ranges between 70% and 90% water. Therefore, all organisms are essentially aqueous systems composed of water and salts derived from these chemicals.

All organisms are made up of macromolecules of these elements, the chemicals being compounded in a highly specific way. Compounded as nucleic acids, they are known as *deoxyribonucleic acid* (DNA), which comprises the genetic information of the organism, and as *ribonucleic acid* (RNA), which is the media by which the DNA information is actualized. As proteins the macromolecules act as catalysts, initiating, speeding up, or strengthening chemical reactions, and as structural components. Bonded as polysaccharides and lipids, these macromolecules are a source of energy and also form structural components. Many sequences and patterns of biochemical reactions are invariant: they always occur in a particular way. Following are a few examples of these timeless constancies:

- Anaerobic glycolysis, a kind of fermentation process in which the potential energy residing in polysaccharides is activated during such functions as muscle contraction
- Citric acid cycle, a circuitous transformation series engineered by a finely integrated set of enzymes located in the mitochondrion, a cell organelle. The cycle serves to generate new energy, largely in the form of high-energy phosphate bonds, as each reaction in the cycle culminates.

Table 1–1.
A Cue to Biologic Holism: the Basic Biochemical Schema of all Terrestrial Organisms

Chemical Element	Biologic Function
A. *Invariant Components:*	
Hydrogen	Required by all organisms for synthesis of organic compounds
Carbon	
Nitrogen	
Oxygen	
Sulfur	
B. *Important Elements Which Are Abundant in Nature:*	
Sodium	Major extracellular cation
Potassium	Major intracellular cation
Chloride	Predominant extracellular and intracellular anion
Calcium	Cofactor of enzymes, important structural element in membranes and bones
Magnesium	Cofactor of enzymes, important to the activation of intracellular energy transfer
Phosphorus	Centrally involved in synthesis of organic compounds, energy transfer
C. *Critical trace elements:*	
Cobalt	Part of vitamin B_{12} complex, important in maturation of red blood cells
Copper	Cofactor of oxidative enzymes
Iodine	Component of thyroxine, therefore, important to body metabolism
Iron	Vital to oxidative processes, enzymes
Manganese	Cofactor of special enzymes
Zinc	Cofactor in many enzymes, important in tissue healing, growth

- Nucleic acid replication and transcription of genetic information
- Protein biosynthesis
- Fatty acid biosynthesis[5]

Nearly every chemical action in the body is controlled by enzymes. Enzymes appear to have a very special relation to time, for the effectiveness of enzymes over simple inorganic catalysts is said to be on the order of 10^8 to 10^9 (*i.e.*, 100,000,000 to 1,000,000,000) times faster. It is enzyme synthesis, to a significant degree, that determines how energy will be utilized for the vital metabolism of the organism and that regulates the rate of the organism's reaction to this energy. Consequently, it is the enzymes that account for the high degree of organization seen in the living process.

The input of energy itself into living systems is also consistent. The flow of energy through the organism has been found to be channeled primarily through the synthesis, storage, and utilization of high-energy phosphate bonds. The basic patterns of this flow are the same throughout the range of aerobic microorganisms to the higher plants and animals and to humans. The structural plan of the mitochondrion, the site of generation of new energy into the cell, is similar in all organisms. This is true regardless of the origin of the tissue or of the species from which the specimen is taken.

These consistencies give us a base for the cognizance that life is a highly controlled holistic process. It would seem that it is because humans have such an immense capacity for control that they remain masters of their fate to the large extent that appears to be the case. This constraint is many faceted, for chemical, electrical, informational, molecular, spatial, and field control are all acknowledged. Nevertheless, even the mere recognition of the multidimensionality of the constraint provides some direction to the search for the key to the organization underlying the many patterns of energy interplay intrinsic to the life process. These patterns belie a wholeness to the conception of life as we know it.

The Modern Philosophical Basis of Holism

Strangely, it was a person uninvolved with biologic theory, Jan Smuts, a South African general, who first took pen in hand in our era to voice conviction that evolution itself demonstrated ". . . a synthetic tendency in the universe" whose underlying patterning indicates ". . . the gradual development and stratification of a progressive series of wholes, stretching from the inorganic beginnings to the highest levels of spiritual creation." He gave the term *holism* to this mode of conceptualization.[6]

The Contemporary Paradigm Shift: Prigogine's Theory of Dissipative Structures in Open Systems

It is only now, several decades after Smuts' proposal, that substantive theory based on mathematical proof has begun to demonstrate for us the elegance of his idea. Since the nineteenth century, physical theory and all Western thought have held to a conception that all organized matter, that is, all information, must degrade. This idea, called *entropy*, was built upon a mechanistic modeling fostered in the age of the Industrial Revolution when it seemed obvious that machines could not refuel or regenerate themselves over time. This conception took the form of a law, the Second Law of Thermodynamics, which was thought to be inviolable and to be the case for all matter, animate as well as inanimate. However, in our time a Belgian physical chemist, Ilya Prigogine, won the Nobel Prize for his confrontation of the question: How can order be derived from entropy? This question had evaded answer by the foremost thinkers of the last century. Prigogine's answer was almost judo-like in that his strategy was to use the strength of the opponent, in this case the Second Law of Thermodynamics, against itself.

Basically, Prigogine's theory states that in all open systems order in nature emerges as a natural concomitant of entropy itself. He calls the energy forms in open systems "dissipative structures," for he states that they can dissipate or "dump" their entropy into the environment with which they interact.

Living beings have been at the base of concern of physicists and biologists alike, for the life process with its ability to be self-organizing and self-regulating has been a major exception to the physics of the Second Law of Thermodynamics. Prigogine's theory states that in all dissipative structures a self-organizing pattern is formed. This pattern is maintained by a continuous dynamic flow which, because of dynamism, becomes increasingly complex. In Prigogine's modeling it becomes evident that with the increased complexity there is a simultaneous increase in the energy that must be dissipated or expended for the maintenance of the structure because it is in constant flux. This state of flux makes the open system very unstable and, therefore, liable to sudden change. These shifts can be numerous and, if they reach a critical state, the effects can be amplified as system interacts with system. Because each system may have numerous energetic connectivities, the synergistic effect can thrust the dynamic forces involved toward a new state. Prigogine theorizes, on the basis of mathematical proof, that this new state may be characterized by greater order, coherence, and connectivity, and, therefore, may exhibit an increased diversification or complexity.

Prigogine's theory squarely confronts the Second Law of Thermodynamics and, as he says, ". . . yields a new scientific intuition about the nature of our universe."[7] Its power is that it gives us a new conceptual view and therefore a new language in which to frame questions about the nature of the universe.

Prigogine's conception of open systems as dissipating structures has shattered the chain of mechanistic theory that has pervaded fundamental Western thinking for over a century. It has replaced it with one that is more in consonance with a holistic world view. His theory has been found applicable to such diverse fields as biology, behavioral psychology, astrophysics, sociology, and economics. Prigogine himself has said:

> I believe in the essential unity of culture. For instance, you can see manifestations of similar ideas at the beginning of the century in the reformulation of space–time by Einstein, the reformulation of music by Schönberg and the reformulation of painting by Cezanne.

The Brain as a Hologram

The paradigm shift stimulated by Prigogine's theory of dissipating structures gives new evidence of the essential unity of culture in reference to the very theme of holism. Karl Pribram, an eminent neuroscientist at Stanford University, and David Bohm, a theoretical physicist at Birkbeck College, London University, have both reformulated our current ideas about reality in a manner that lends additional credence to holistic concepts about the way the universe works.

Pribram's research in neurology led him to believe that the brain's deep structures were analogous to a hologram. For instance, specific memory is not confined to a particular locus but rather, based on the work of neurologist Karl Lashley, memory seems to be distributed throughout the brain. As a young scientist Pribram worked with Lashley and had been impressed not only that memory was distributed throughout the brain in encoded form, but also that the code incorporated the whole of the memory. He thought of the analogy of the hologram, for in the hologram any piece of the holographic plate will reconstruct the entirety of the image.

The hologram was first described by Dennis Gabor in 1947, but it was not constructed (by Leith and Upatnicks) until the discovery of the coherent light known as the laser beam about 15 years later.[8] In holography, a photographic plate records as an interference pattern the field of light that is scattered by an object. This plate, the hologram, is then exposed to a coherent light, such as the laser beam, where the light wave phases are matched as they are emitted. Upon such exposure the entire original wave pattern, or image, can be seen in three dimensions in the hologram, each perspective being visually correct.

Pribram's idea was that a hologram was created at the interstices of patterned electrical activity as the neurons of the brain were activated.[9] Pressing the logic of his thought, which is based in theoretical mathematics, he envisioned the perception of physical reality by the deep brain structures as a holistic interpretation of wave frequencies "in an invisible matrix that is other than three dimensional."[10]

The Universe as a Hologram

Bohm's conception was that the nature of the universe is essentially a hologram. He says that this reality has ". . . an enfolded order, a cohesive interconnectedness" in which "events," or occurrences, arise to consciousness as frequencies beyond those we recognize as time and space; that is, they are potentially a function of simultaneity.[11] The enfolded order is always whole and is essentially independent of time. However, we use time to make the enfolded order meaningful to our perceptions.

These frequencies that Pribram and Bohm discuss are said to emerge ". . . from an other than three dimensional invisible matrix," a multidimensional matrix of connectivities of interacting wave phenomena that underlie the very stuff of the universe. Individually we begin to recognize these frequencies in the variety of wavelengths at the molecular level of organization of the nutrients we feed our bodies, and in the light, ionization, and sound waves that accompany our interactions with the environment. Therefore, they have direct implications for our *health* (a term that defines the direction of our striving: that is, *heal* from the Middle English *haelen*, and -th, a suffix indicating a state or condition).

The Holistic Nature of Perception

The Psyche

The striving toward health, toward a state of being whole, is a common human aspiration. The problem is that humans are sentient as well as physical beings, and from that perspective each of us seems to be two beings, or to reflect two images. One image is turned toward and immersed in concerns about one's relationship to the external world with its responsibilities, duties, and rituals. The other being is concerned with the actualization of one's interior self, one's essential being.

The bridge between these realms is called the *psyche*. It can be considered as a space within each person that is either symbolic or real. It is the "place" where images and feeling tones may be loosely bound during surges or wellings-up of instinctive knowledge and where they act together in an attempt to give each of us a "working knowledge" of ourselves as human beings.[12] If this knowledge leads us to achieve emotional fulfillment in life and to perfect (or complete) ourselves as feeling, living beings, we may be said to have achieved psychodynamic wholeness.[13] This achievement is not frequent in our culture because the realm of the psyche is, in fact, the domain of the unconscious. The unconscious has only recently begun to be understood within a modern frame of reference.

The Unconscious

It is thought that human consciousness has developed by specific steps or evolution from mysterious beginnings in the unconscious. It is through the functional development of consciousness that humans have been enabled to gradually free themselves from the primal grip of nature and to exert some individual and volitional freedom.[14] Nevertheless, it is the unconscious which is the depository or ground state of human experience. Because it reaches so far back into humanity's early history (literally defining humanness), it controls or determines the individual's life in ways that are unapparent or mysterious. Translated into terms of the psyche, it is this spectrum of meaningfulness that arises out of the primordial matrices of life experience to span the farther reaches of abstract thought, the unique mind-stuff of humans. It is here that is reflected the ". . . enfolded order, a cohesive interconnectedness" which arises from ". . . frequencies in an invisible matrix that is other than three-dimensional." The holographic analogue can be conceptualized because it is experienced.

The Use of Myth

The intellectual grasp of the holistic nature of human perception of the universe, however, had its root beginnings in less abstract modes of thinking. Our culture's best guesses about how early men and women viewed reality is through the reflections of mythic imagery and symbolism. It was (and is) through the acting out of mythic themes that human beings participate in that reality; that is, we become contemporary with that myth and experientially understand it.[15]

Myths are written in symbolic language, a symbolism that is awesomely similar the world over because mythic images do not belong to one culture but rather to all. The same mythic themes arise in even geographically removed cultures, no matter how far apart they are, and therefore seem to be a hallmark of the human condition. Because of this universality, the interpretation of reality through metaphor embedded in these transcultural myths appears to be a function of being human. This trait comes down through time to the contemporary era in common and homely ways for, as Warren Hemp (Temple University) has remarked, in modern man the right hemisphere of the brain and the language of the body continue to speak to us metaphorically.

Interestingly, it can also be said that in the following ways myth is in a sense similar to science:

- It attempts to give a unified and consistent explanation of nature and make it intelligible.
- It attempts to influence nature and universal events.
- It recognizes that it only "approximates the truth."

Although dreams use mythic figures and appear to strive toward holism also, there are significant differences which authorities on the matter, such as Eliade, are careful to note.[16] Through studies in comparative religion, ethnology, and Oriental philosophy it is known that the myth is characteristic of man in archaic and ancient societies. On the other hand, dreams are most characteristic of man in modern societies that are built upon the Western model. It is said that evidence for this assumption presents itself to us through depth psychology and the systematic study of symbolism. Eliade makes the distinction that, whereas myths concern themselves with interpretations of the mysteries of human behavior and of reality and are based on a universal model, dreams are personal and private interpretations that may not conform to reality. Nevertheless, the mythic base continues to be reborn in the dreams, fantasies, and yearnings of modern man, although the realization may lie fallow in the more remote depths of the psyche.

Myths have great power during times of crises and decision. As myths gain structure they frequently become ritualized and form the basis of sacred traditions. These traditions lay the foundations for exemplary patterns of human behavior that eventually become codified in the social structure. Within the social structure they form the basis of instruction in initiatory rites or other forms of education and become part of the cultural tradition, part of the way humans remember.

The Translation Through Symbol

The memory of myth translates itself through symbol, the figurative or metaphoric language of the psyche. In effect, the symbol is an objective, unitary expression of several ideas whose composite meaning is usually profound and difficult to define. Early in the primitive development of social structure at the bare dawn of prehistory the symbol of woman appears. Survival itself is based on the fertility of women and, therefore, it can be understood why the most ancient figurines, statuettes, and symbolic pictographs and cave paintings to be found have been those concerned with fertility rites.

The Feminine Principle

It would seem that a direct proportion existed between the rate of infant mortality in a tribe or clan and the importance of a fertility cult in the social structure. Quite universally (as now, for instance, in the

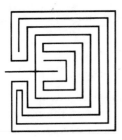 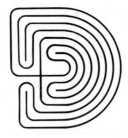

Fig. 1–1.
Two types of the Mother Earth symbol of the Hopis. The whole myth and meaning of the Emergence (of the present fourth world) are expressed by one symbol known to the Hopis as the Mother Earth symbol. *(Redrawn from Waters F: Book of the Hopi. New York, Ballantine Books, 1974)*

tantric yoga system) the moon goddess was thought to be the ruler of fertility. This notion has a factual base in the lunar cycling of the menstrual period and the duration of pregnancy. The crescent shape reminiscent of the lunar phases became the symbol of the feminine principle, which was later enlarged to signify the unconscious or instinctive state as well.

As social structuring matured, it was through the exploration of the feminine role that early men and women began to realize the importance of intimacy and touch and mutual support. The mother's attentiveness to her child and her tenderness in its care became a training ground for human psychological development. A mother's love, her indulgence of childish foibles, and her understanding, forgiveness, and protection are unforgettable memories that mark each person. Therefore, in most people mother symbols tend to evoke a sense of awe or arouse feelings of devotion.

Jung has discussed the infinite number of aspects that have been assigned to the conceptualization of the mother figure,[17] and notes that these qualities may hold either positive or negative connotations. The more affirmative qualities include maternal solicitude and sympathy, any helpful instinct or impulse, and all that fosters growth and fertility and is benign and sustaining. In addition, of a more spirited and decisive nature are attributes of magical authority, wisdom, and ".... spiritual exaltation that transcends reason." Counter to these are qualities that are secretive and hidden, situations that are ". . . terrifying and inescapable, like fate," and concerns about the world of the dead. Jung notes that the symbolic influence of the mother figure may induce humaneness, compassion, and wisdom in children by fostering qualities of tenderness, concern for enduring values, strong religious feelings, sensitive responses to intuitive knowledge, and curiosity about the riddles of the universe.

Looking back over this list of attributes, one begins to understand a natural evolution of the role of the nurse as the result of a maturing expression of the feminine principle in both men and women, because all children may grow up with strong female–maternal identifications. Although in the past males have been forcibly removed from this climate of female concern by masculine rites of passage at puberty, there has been a decided effort in our present era to allow the male greater freedom in the exploration of the feminine principle to which both sexes are heir.

For the female of our species the understanding and acting out of the feminine principle is more natural because of her active role in the bearing and rearing of children and because of her traditional task of caring for those in the family unit who are helpless or dying. Over time, these humane concerns foster a deepening knowledge of natural modes of healing and helping that can be quite direct and innovative.

References

1. Whitehead AN: Science and the Modern World, pp 9–10. New York, The New American Library, 1953
2. Capra F: The Tao of Physics, pp 25, 203, 287–307. Berkeley, Shambhala, 1975
3. Nillson L: Behold Man, pp 49–56. Boston, Little, Brown, 1973
4. Handler P (ed): Biology and the Future of Man, p 66. London, Oxford University Press, 1970
5. Kenyon DH, Steinman G: Biochemical Predestination, p 4. New York, McGraw-Hill, 1969
6. Smuts J: Holism and Evolution. New York, Macmillan, 1926 (particularly pp 82–83, 86–87, 188–119, 314, 337–345)
7. Browne MW: Scientist sees loophole in physical law. New York Times, pp C1, C3, May 29, 1979
8. Leith E, Upatnicks J: Photography by laser. Sci Am pp 24–35, June, 1965
9. Pribram K: How is it that sensing so much we can do so little? In Schmitt FD, Worden FG (eds): The Neurosciences, III. New York, The Rockefeller Press, 1974
10. Brain/Mind Bulletin 2(16), July 4, 1977 (entire issue)
11. Brain/Mind Bulletin, *Loc cit*
12. Progoff I: The Symbolic and the Real, p 104. New York, McGraw-Hill, 1963
13. Durckheim KG: A practice to achieve man's wholeness, Part II. Image 64:3, 1974
14. Neumann E: The Origins and History of Consciousness. Translated by RFC Hull. Princeton, Princeton University Press (Bollingen Series XLII), 1954
15. Eliade M: Myths, Dreams and Mysteries, p 31 (English language edition). New York, Harpers Torchbook, 1960
16. Eliade, *op cit*, pp 7–8
17. Jung CG: Four Archetypes, pp 7–44. Translated by RFC Hull. Princeton, Princeton University Press (Bollingen Series XX), 1973

2 Holistic Health in Primitive Cultures: Shamanism

Shamanism as a Feminine Role

Women's imperative of caring for the ill and injured within the family of necessity sharpened their healing skills. Family shamanism arose as a natural development, with women in the predominant roles.[1] Shamanism, a form of ecstatic healing in which the practitioner is in a heightened state of consciousness, is said to go back to the Upper Paleolithic period.[2] Murphy, in discussing the feminine role in shamanism, says that female shamanism preceded male shamanism. He documents the cultural history as follows:[3]

- Almost all women shamanized at least by the time of their old age.
- With the passage of time the role of shaman was shared by both male and female adults.
- Within the more recent historical times a crystallization of the shamanic role into a more professional stance took place and the position required considerable talent and stylized training.

Over time the shaman's role expanded to that of healer, seer, and visionary, to what Rothenberg has poetically named "technician of the sacred."[4]

It is not surprising that women were the first to play the role of shaman. Besides having ample opportunity to practice on their own families, women had considerable power in decision-making because early culture was matrilineal. It was the women who were in charge of the cultural mores; they saw to it that the community continued to follow the natural ways.[5] Among the *Han de no san nee*, the Six Nations People, the formation of the nuclear family was advocated, and the culture of the People of the Longhouse emphasized fidelity within the marriage relationship. Out of this background, women, with the natural abilities inherent in the playing out of the feminine principle as noted in Chapter 1, easily assumed the role of shaman.

Shamanism as an Enactment of the Feminine Principle

Evidence of the close linkage of shamanism with the feminine principle has been noted even in recent historical accounts of shamanism. For instance, among the Chuckee in Siberia, there is a long tradition of feminization of male initiates into what has been called "a soft man being" to enhance their shamanistic abilities.[6,7] One can see how this need arose among a people whose survival depended on the hunting of the great beasts, because in an encounter of such heroic proportions the hunter needed some means of foretelling the outcome of the encounter. Forewarned was forearmed. Therefore, in many of these ancient cultures adolescent youths were encouraged to hallucinate because visions were part of the accepted ways of acquiring information.[8] Persons sensitive to dreams, telepathy, or the sensing of invisible presences that resulted in premonition or omen were highly regarded.

The Call to Shamanship

Similar to contemporary times, shamanship in the past occurred in several ways:

- The role was taken on as a spontaneous choice by the individual, either as a special calling or by selection or election of the tribe or the clan.
- The role was acquired through hereditary transmission, either genetic or through a mother or father figure.
- The role was acquired by personal decision based on individual motivation.
- An individual accepted the role in response to the will of the clan.

This last manner of attaining shamanship through community insistence could occur because, although the chief function of the shaman was healing, in most ethnic societies shamans were also involved in other magico-religious rites that affected the welfare of the group. These included rain-making, the harvesting of crops, and hunting. Jung notes that their prophetic dreams often were archetypal and contained a world vision or a cosmic truth. Shamans were highly valued for this ability.

Simultaneity of Shamanic Practices Among Different Cultures

Shamanic practices are worldwide, extending from the Arctic vastness of Siberia (where Rasputin was a renowned shaman) to the far reaches of Tierra del Fuego. One can see how homely remedies and practices could become encapsulated in ritual upon which social structures depend for their continuation. For instance, a Stone Age people, the Tasaday, were found in the early 1960s to be living deep in the jungles of the Philippine Islands under seemingly untouched primitive conditions.[9] Unlike modern birthing practices which are surrounded by medical technological procedures, the Tasaday do not cut the umbilical cord immediately after a child is born. Rather, after the delivery of her child, the mother is given a drink made from a locally growing flower. The chemical constituents of the concoction help speed the separation of the placenta. It is only after the placenta has been expelled that the umbilical cord is cut between placenta and child. The placenta is then buried at the base of a tree, which to the Tasaday (as well as to their more modern counterparts, ourselves) is symbolic of growth and age (the tree of life). After the birth of the child, the mother is given the liver of a wild animal to eat. The modern counterpart of this in Western societies is the iron supplements given new mothers to counteract the iron depletion of the mother's body that frequently occurs during pregnancy.

Women among other primitive societies have many opportunities to learn in a first-hand manner of the healthful qualities of natural foods that may be used to promote healing. Inupiat (Eskimo) women, with children in tow, forage the tundra and hillsides for edibles. They comb the waterfowl breeding grounds for the eggs of cranes, loons, geese, and swans. In addition to eating the yolk and the albumin, they crush the shells of these eggs for a calcium source for their families. They gather tender summer greens and marinate them in seal oil and keep these vitamin-laden nutrients for use during the dark Arctic winter months. Inupiat women are frequently left at home while their men go hunting, and during such times their main entertainment is visiting among each other. Since discussion of life experiences occupies much of the time during such visits, these women become quite proficient psychotherapists as well.

Faced as they are with a harsh environment that allows them limited conditions for travel, Inupiat women are forced to use their own ingenuity in times of stress. Delia, a lady "Eskimo doctor" whom I met above the Arctic Circle in Alaska, demonstrated to me a simple and elegant technique she developed for disengaging a child who is in breech position for delivery or who has the umbilical cord around its neck, without any danger to either mother or child. While the mother is in a sitting position, Delia sits directly facing the mother, close enough for the inner aspects of her lower arms to be on either side of the mother's swollen abdomen. She then brings her arms to within an inch or two of the mother's abdomen. With a rhythmic series of flicks of her wrists, done in such a manner that both hands and forearms are alternately turned (so that the inner aspects are turned uppermost and just touch the abdomen) and returned to the normal position, Delia gently makes a rhythmic contact with the mother's abdomen. This serves to put the amniotic fluid into a series of wavelike motions. The continuous eddies of the disturbed amniotic fluid serve also to move the fetus from its position and, Delia says, ". . . . it just floats up toward the top of its mama's belly." With great sensitivity of touch Delia feels the mother's abdomen for the pulsation of the umbilical arteries to assure herself that the umbilical cord floats free in the womb, and checks the mother frequently thereafter.

The Underlying Holism of the Ancient Ways

As one studies ancient ways, time and again one is faced by the fact that holism reaches deeply into the natural perception of the universe. The Native Americans again provide an example. Their languages always emphasize modes of interrelatedness of their ideas about the universe, so that the speaker never loses sight of an ultimate wholeness. They consider human beings to be microcosms of the universe, and even their traditional dwelling places are modeled on their conceptions of the process of the creation of the world.[10] They see a continuum of life energy in every object, inanimate as well as animate. Luther Standing Bear, a contemporary Lakota Sioux, states it well:

> But very early in life the child began to realize that wisdom was all about and everywhere and that there were many things to know. There was no such thing as emptiness in the world. Even in the sky there were no vacant places. Everywhere there was life visible and invisible and every object gave us a great interest in life. Even without human companionship one was never alone. The world teemed with life and wisdom, there was no complete solitude for the Lakota.[11]

With this view of the cosmos, to the Native American the symbol is actually considered to be the same as that to which it refers, its meaning being intuitively grasped. For instance, the anthropologist Brown notes that when a Navaho singer does a sandpainting of a god, it is not considered that the sandpainting simply represents the god, but rather that the god is actually present in the painting and directly casts its power and grace upon all those participating in the ceremony. One would think that this is symbolically similar in manner to the religious act of transubstantiation among Catholics. A presence is also believed to be actualized when an Apache or Navaho singer invokes a deity or chants a mythic event; then ".... the reality of the action or the event is neither of the past nor of the future, but of the moment, the *now* of mythic time."[12]

The Sandpainting as Mandala

In reference to the sandpainting, the mandala is constructed around the concept of the interdependence and integration in time of all phenomena through their unitive relationship with the one eternal center, the focus of one's being, the matrix of all events. The sandpainting, therefore, is a kind of mandala of healing. The term *mandala* is derived from the Sanskrit and means *circle*. The mandala is concerned with circular images, which can be drawn, painted, modeled, or danced, as happens in the Dervish monasteries. It was introduced into the world of Western psychotherapy largely through the work of C.G. Jung. In studying the accounts of his patients, Jung found that they frequently referred to mandalas (although they didn't know them to be such) which appeared spontaneously in dreams, during certain states of conflict, and in the imagery of schizophrenics.

Mandalas are also used within a religious context as an aid to contemplation and to promote spiritual growth. As such they may be seen in the monasteries of the Roman Catholic Church as well as in Buddhist lamaseries, particularly those of Tibetan Buddhism. The use of the mandala reaches quite far back in history, perhaps to paleolithic times as seen in Zimbabwe, Africa in certain rock paintings of the sun wheel (Fig. 2–1).

As we understand it today, the purpose of the mandala is twofold: (1) to delimit or clear a space where the individual will be safe and (2)

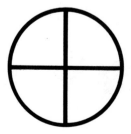

Fig. 2–1.
The sun wheel.

to produce a magic circle in which a person's sickness will be healed through a supernatural act of the supreme deity who is identified with or enshrined in the center of the mandala. The power of the mandala is therefore in its center. This is so whether we are talking about Navaho sandpaintings or Tibetan Buddhist mandalas.

In Tibetan Buddhism the mandala is used as a *yantra*, a tool to assist meditation or concentration. At the center is usually either the image of the most sublime of the religious figures appropriate to the occasion or the image of a *dorje*, the symbol of a thunderbolt, which stands for unlimited power and its control. Father Sky and Mother Earth are depicted in the Navaho sandpaintings. Symbols of pollen and cornmeal—both life-sustaining staples—or symbols of thunderbolts are also used. There are many Christian mandalas, one of which is of Christ Triumphant surrounded by the symbols of the four evangelists, the bull, the eagle, the lion, and the angel. Another mandala has come down to us through the Egyptians and is seen on the back of a United States one-dollar bill. It is an eye enclosed in a triangle (Fig. 2–2), a mandala which today is thought of as an abstract design representing a spiritual or supernatural experience, the structure of the eye representing the center of order of the unconscious which is held together by the protective triangle. This is also a Christian symbol representing the all-seeing eye of God in the Trinity.

The mandala, therefore, can be considered a paradigm or model of the psyche. The Jungian interpretation is that the working out of the mandala represents a quest for the center of the personality, a focal point within the psyche ". . . where everything is related and by which everything is arranged and which is itself a source of energy." Crossculturally this spontaneous holistic act can have considerable therapeutic effect. In the case of the sandpainting, the sandpainting is constructed step by step and the ill person is led or carried step by step to the center of the sandpainting in a manner somewhat analogous to the Christian enactment of the Stations of the Cross.

The self-healing quality of the mandala was described in a personal communication between Jung and a Tibetan Buddhist abbot. The latter said mandalas were models for the active imagination. If a person in a lamasery had a religious conflict or a critical personal

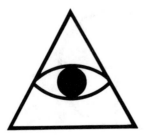

Fig. 2–2.
A mandala. This symbol has been used by the Ancient Egyptians, by Christians, and by the United States government.

problem, that person built a mandala, entered into it in meditation, and worked out a solution to the conflict.[13] In such a case we can see that it is the active concentration of the individual that induces the reintegration. With sandpainting reintegration occurs in the patient through answering questions put by the shaman, by the imaginal figures suggested by the chant, or by other involvement in the ceremony which requires concentration and participation (Fig. 2–3). In essence the technique is judo-like in that one uses the psychic forces by which one is bound to a situation and, in a highly controlled fashion, consciously uses the energy of these constellated images against themselves and so transcends them.

The mandala thus is seen as an instinctive act toward self-healing. Within the Jungian conception, therefore, the mandala can lead to an emergence of self, of the essential being of the individual. With this emergence a new energy is introduced into the reach of the individual psyche, and a rebirth or transformation occurs.

The Realms of the Medicine Man and of the Shaman

Among the native North Americans illnesses were thought to be of two kinds: those that were due to pathogenic agents and those that were the consequences of "soul loss." A medicine man or woman or other healing person could treat the former; only a shaman could treat the latter. This was because it was recognized that, whereas the visionary experience was a natural potential in all people, it was only the shaman with his or her special relationship to the spirit lives who was able to enter deeply into the supernatural world and retrieve the lost soul of the ill person.[14] This was of vital importance to the society, for the religious rituals concerned the experiences of the human soul, and the soul might be open to assault by demons and sorcerers who might inflict harm on the individual.

Illnesses considered to be due to soul loss were caused by flight of the soul, by outright possession of the soul by evil beings, by the placement of a magical object into the ill person's body, or by frightening dreams during which the soul strayed.[15] Descriptions of symptoms in these categories are of interest since they can be related to the malfunctioning of the autonomic nervous system. Weakness, loss of appetite, fainting, dizziness, fear, feelings of suffocation, feelings of futility, confusion, and frightening dreams are some symptoms that are mentioned. Recovery from these maladies is indication of the restoration of balance in the ill person, so that healing is a holistic act.

The shaman uses methods of concentration, abstinence from both food and sex, chemicals such as hallucinogenic cacti and peyote (this among the Native Americans; shamans in other parts of the world use indigenous substances), and trance-like states of consciousness.

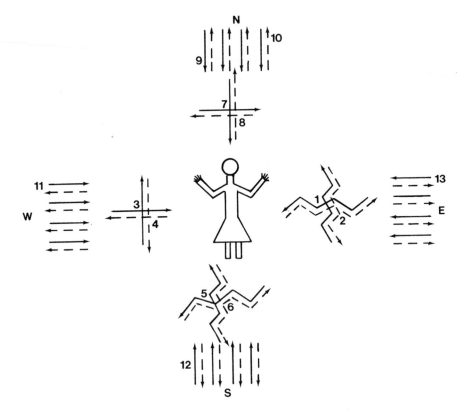

Fig. 2-3.
Ritualistic acts of Restoration rite: Shooting Chant. Restoration is a rite of every ceremony; it restores to normal a person who has been shocked or frightened into unconsciousness. The Restoration symbol looks something like a crank; in the Shooting Chant it represents a straight lightening. Instructions: **Step 1:** with a tail-feathered arrow mark two crossed zigzag lightenings in the sand at the east toward the patient. **Step 2:** erase 1 with foot away from patient. **Step 3:** make two straight lightenings crossed at the west toward the patient. **Step 4:** erase 3 with foot away from patient. **Step 5:** make same drawing as 1 at south toward the patient. **Step 6:** erase 5 away from patient. **Step 7:** make same drawing as 3 at north toward patient. **Step 8:** erase 7 away from patient. **Step 9:** make four small straight lines at north toward patient. **Step 10:** erase 9 away from patient. **Step 11:** repeat 9 and 10 at west. **Step 12:** repeat 9 and 10 at south. **Step 13:** repeat 9 and 10 at east (note anti-sunwise circuit). **Step 14:** press patient at ceremonial points. **Step 15:** incensing: 2 coals. *(Redrawn from Reichard A: Navaho Religion. Princeton, Princeton University Press, 1974)*

Sometimes natural functions such as sleep are used to establish a means of communication with the spirits so that an illness can be cured.[16] In the case of soul loss, attaining an ecstatic state, one of the methods learned at initiation, seems to be universally employed by shamans to "overtake" the soul.[17]

Another universal trait of shamanic healing seems to be that its practices are uniquely individualistic both in regard to the shaman's relationship with his or her spirit helpers or spirit guardians and in reference to the experience of the healee during the healing ceremony. In the shamanic relationship to the spirits it is usually the shaman who controls the spirits; that is, it is not a case of direct possession in which the shaman becomes a mere instrument of the helping spirit. It is a conjoint action usually built on cooperation. The fact that there are both generalized commonalities as well as individualistically recognized marks of shamanism cues us that there must be underlying, although as yet unrecognized, universal laws of nature which shape these behaviors.

There is a myth found in several parts of the world of a road of the gods that reaches between the earth and the sky. This road is frequently represented by the rainbow and is seen in such figures as the ziggurat of Babylonia. The shaman in search of assistance by the gods travels this rainbow bridge seeking the soul of the ill person. This is made possible through the resonance of the shaman's drum, which is played as an accompaniment as the shaman attains the ecstatic state. Again, quite universally, this ecstatic state or magical flight is represented by a feather. Among the Native North Americans the flight is represented by the eagle feather.

The Underlying Basis of Life Energy

As an example of common shamanic beliefs about the basic life factor in human beings, one could look to the studies of Meyerhoff[18] and other anthropologists who have studied the shamans of MesoAmerica. Among the Huichal (who call themselves the Wixárika) in the Sierra Madre country of Mexico, the fundamental life force is called *kupüri** and relates to the soul or the consciousness, for it is said " . . . it lives in the (crown of) the head . . . where we think." This energy, *kupüri*, is described in considerable detail and in terms so graphic that one can easily imagine the experience. The *kupüri* is said to be very small—". . . small as a little bug, a fly or a tick"—and emits "a high-frequency

---

*Called kópavi in Hopi. See Walters F: Book of the Hopi, p 16. New York, Ballantine Books, 1963

hissing or whistling sound." When the shaman is seeking the soul that has strayed from the body of an ill person, he or she listens intently during the search. When the shaman hears the distinctive sound of the *kupüri,* communication is made by the shaman whistling to it or making a hissing sound said to resemble the sputtering of a fire fed by wood that is not completely dry. These mimicries of natural sounds attract the *kupüri.* The shaman then helps it retrace its path to the body that belongs to it. This is done by following the thin filament, which is ". . . like spider's silk" by which each individual is connected to his or her *kupüri* from the crown of the head. It is said that if this life essence spills out from the top of the head, it will result in death. We shall see that these ideas and others that are to follow are also held by geographically widely disparate people, such as the yogin of the East.

Current Shamanic Practices

Kaplan and Johnson have studied the psychopathology of the Navaho in the southwestern United States. They quote Father Bernard Haile's description of the Navahos conception of the soul that he wrote when he was a missionary among them. All life, they say, is twofold, having an inner and an outer shell-like form. The outer aspect lives in a state similar to Plato's world of illusion, for its acts and its goals are controlled in actuality by its individual inner form. The latter is in fact the wind-soul, for it is within the wind that we have life, it is the wind that breathes and moves and has speech, thought, and dreams.

There are seven winds in the wind-soul, which are named white, blue, yellow, dark, small, left-handed, and glossy. When these winds are in the correct order or sequence, the person is in a state of well-being. When, however, there is malalignment among the winds, the person will be met by intense, often vicious ill will and may become the victim of witchcraft. The winds are deeply embedded in the personality of the person. They enter the individual at birth and bestow upon the body life energies that greatly influence the individual's personality development.[19]

Many of the ancient therapeutic practices of the Native Americans continue to be used by modern therapists in holistic health practices. Notable among these are massage, sweat baths, sunbathing, counterirritation, local pressure using both hands and feet, and the use of oils. The American Indians also had considerable knowledge about the use of herbs as pharmaceuticals, about the setting of fractures, and what we today would call dentistry. Pre-Columbian South Americans manufactured artificial limbs and false teeth and had expertise in delivering difficult births by what we today call cesarean section.

In 1972 the National Institute of Mental Health announced the financing of the Rough Rock Demonstration School in Arizona because the Institute was convinced that the healing traditions of the Native Americans had validity and should be supported and sustained. The trainees were reported to have cured facial tics, partial paralysis, dizzy spells, insomnia, and schizophrenia under controlled tests and supervision.[20]

In addition to chants, sandpainting, and other ceremonial rituals, the students learned the therapuetic use of 150 to 200 pharmaceutical herbs. These medicinals work, it is said, because of the divinity imbued in the herbs, acting to restore the unity of the individual. Other modern shamans feel that some diseases are beyond the ability of the shaman to heal. These are called "White man's diseases." Included among such diseases are ulcers, cirrhosis of the liver, and certain cancers.[21]

The therapies of the shaman strike deeply into the psyche. Halifax describes the effect of the shaman song as follows: "The song word is powerful; it names a thing, it stands at the sacred center, drawing all towards it . . . The word disappears, the poetry is gone, but the imaginal form persists within the mind and works on the soul."[22]

Another powerful psychotherapeutic tool is public confession. Among the Western Apache the confession is voluntary and not a prerequisite of healing. Nevertheless, before treatment is given the shaman may refer tangentially to the patient's past by asking, "Have you done anything bad?" This ploy is in alignment with the most sophisticated theories of modern psychosomatic therapeutics.[23]

Indeed, confession as a psychotherapeutic technique among shamans has been called "virtually a pan-American trait." Radin described the effect of the peyote ceremony as threefold: hallucinatory exhilaration, vomiting (and therefore cathartic), and verbal confession. Describing the peyote ceremony of the Winnebago at the turn of the twentieth century, he said that by about midnight " . . . the peyote begins to affect some people. These generally rise and deliver self-accusatory speeches, after which they go around shaking hands with everyone, asking for forgiveness."[24] This tradition continues today. In a tenuous fashion it is somewhat reminiscent of the group therapies of the early 1970s.

Among the Iglulik Eskimos, illnesses thought to be due to the violation of sacred taboos were treated through collective confession. At the insistence of the shaman, who uses "spirit language," each of the members of the family or group one after the other openly confessed his or her sins or transgressions.[25] This sense of collective responsibility for a group member's illness has yet to be replicated in Western civilizations, except perhaps for a sense of group responsibility for environmental carcinogens.

In sum, the pattern that presents itself is that the shaman's approach is essentially holistic. The shaman is primarily concerned with the removal of the healee's symptoms. He or she devises overt and covert means whereby the healee can be relieved of conditions of stress and the suffering of intense emotional pain and their psychosomatic sequelae. The shaman also engages in considerable symbolic and practical counseling, creating positive, expectant attitudes and encouraging a sense of responsibility for self.

The shaman's entry to shamanism often occurs during a spiritual crisis brought on by a supernatural apparition (of an animal, *e.g.*, a wolf) as a sign or by an "initiatory illness" which may be both severe and debilitating. This is a rite of passage, because in the process of healing the novice frequently has the experience of plunging into the deeper realms of his or her consciousness in which the crisis of the illness acts as a stimulus for the occurrence of a transformative experience. The symbolism of this severe crisis has been compared to the act of mystical death, and the return to wellness suggests an intention and willingness to change one's sensitivity to psychodynamic events in others as well as in self. This reminds one very much of Jung's concept of the archetype of the wounded healer, because it happens very frequently that in order to withdraw maleficent spirits from an ill person, the shaman consciously takes these spirits into his or her own body and therefore in the decisive moments of the crisis struggles and endures more than the patient does.

Rappaport and Dent have concluded from a study of 31 Tanzanian shamans of the Waganga tribe that Western therapists can profit much from a study of shamans, medicine men and women, and diviners. They summarize their reasons for this judgment as follows:

- It is the shaman and not the client who defines the problems.
- Shaman and client have grown up in a large kin network and share cultural and religious values.
- The therapy is focused around the shaman's charisma.
- Treatment is based on a folk model which intimately includes the healee's extended family members and thereby eases the reestablishment of community ties from which the healee may have become alienated. This extended family includes the trees, plants, herbs, animals, and spirits, so that there is no need to feel obliged, as we do in the West, to conquer the environment.
- The shaman helps the client look for meaning in his or her illness. Rappaport and Dent compare this to Frankl's concept of the "search for meaning" which underlies his development of Logotherapy which ". . . makes the concept of man into a whole . . . and focuses its attention upon mankind's groping for a higher meaning in life."[26]

- Finally, Rappaport and Dent conclude that sorcery is a matrix for understanding ill will among the living, the hostilities in personal relationships that foster illness.[27]

In this version of therapeutics, primitive as we may think it to be, healing is seen as a deeply psychodynamic process in which one is actively engaged in the discovery and growth of the soul or inner being, in the full (*i.e.*, holistic) actualization of the individual human potential.

References

1. Murphy JM: Psychotherapeutic aspects of shamanism. In Kiev A (ed): Magic, Faith and Healing, p 73. New York, Free Press, 1964
2. Eliade M: Shamanism, pp 503–504. Princeton, Princeton University Press (Bollingen Series LXXVI), 1972
3. Murphy, *loc cit*
4. Rothenberg J: Technicians of the Sacred. Garden City, Doubleday, 1968
5. Akewesasne Notes. SUNY/Buffalo, Program in American Studies 10(5):30, Winter, 1978
6. Borgoras W: The Chuckchee. In Boas F (ed): Jessup North Pacific Expedition, Book 7, pp 450–451. New York, American Museum of Natural History, Vol. II, 1904–1909
7. Eliade, *op cit*, p 352
8. Grimil P (ed): Larouse World Mythology, p 18. London, Paul Hamlyn, 1972
9. Nance J: The Gentle Tasaday. New York, Harcourt, Brace & Jovanovich, 1975
10. Brown JE: Modes of contemplation through actions: North American Indians. Main Currents in Modern Thought (Retrospective Issue) 32(2–5):193, November 17, 1940–November 17, 1975
11. Brown, *op cit*, p 194
12. Brown, *Loc cit*
13. Harding ME: Psychic Energy: Its Source and Its Transformation, 2nd ed, p 391. Princeton, Princeton University Press (Bollingen Series X), 1973
14. Eliade, *op cit*, p 298
15. Eliade, *op cit*, p 301
16. Eliade, *op cit*, p 219
17. Eliade, *op cit*, p 216
18. Meyerhoff BG: Peyote Hunt, pp 20–21. Ithaca, Cornell University Press, 1974
19. Kaplan B, Johnson D: Navaho psychopathology. In Kiev A (ed): Magic, Faith and Healing, pp 205–206. New York, Free Press, 1964
20. Wilford JN: Medicine man successful where science falls short. New York Times, p 20, July 7, 1972
21. Knudlson P: Flora, shaman of the Wintu. Natural History, p 13, May, 1975
22. Halifax J: Shamanic Voices, p 33. New York, EP Dutton, 1979
23. La Barre W: Confession as a cathartic therapy. In Kiev A (ed): Magic, Faith and Healing, p 41. New York, Free Press, 1964

24. Radin P: A sketch of the peyote cult of the Winnebago. Journal of Religious Psychology 7:3, 1914
25. Eliade, *op cit*, pp 60, 289, 296
26. Frankl V: Man's Search for Meaning, pp 151–214. New York, Washington Square Press, 1965
27. Fergusen M: Charisma, friendliness helpful in folk psychotherapy. Brain/ Mind 4, No. 15:1,3,1979

3 The Chinese Sphere of Influence

The central thesis of this book is that there are important cues to universal laws about healthy human functions and behaviors which can be perceived when one impartially examines within a historical perspective humanity's thoughts about the body, emotions, mind, and world. It is suggested that it is the repetitive natural descriptions over vast reaches of time of bodily functions and feeling–thinking behaviors to which one looks for these laws of nature. The underlying assumption here is that the perspective of a person's reflexions on self is molded by the human condition in which he or she is involved. Therefore, the images the person sees and feels are the natural resultants of the working out of these laws of nature.

It has been noted previously that primitive societies, even though they may have been far apart geographically, held beliefs in common about their health functions. As the analysis proceeds through several of the ancient civilizations, it will be noted that there persists a continuity of thought between cultures about how humans relate to nature.

One such concept, which continues to be relevant even in contemporary societies, is the humoral theory. According to this ancient theory, the body contains certain humors, health being the result of the proper balance of these humors and disease being the result of their imbalance. Today the humoral theory is believed to be related to different body types and their characteristic susceptibilities to certain illnesses. In the representative ancient civilizations described here, these humors have a decided consistency, although they may be stated variously.

According to the ancient Chinese, there were (and continue to be) six humors based upon the fundamental life energy, *ch'i*. In the individual the *ch'i* is conditioned by the polarizing *yin* and *yang* energies so that the qualitative states of health are ordered into opposite characteristics: hot—cold, wet—dry, heavy—light, male—female, dark—bright, strong—weak, active—congested, and so on. In the Ayurvedic system of ancient India there were (and continue to be) three humors:

phlegm (*kapha*), bile (*pitta*), and wind (*vayu*). The derivative systems that originated in the Mediterranean area noted four humors: yellow bile, black bile, phlegm, and blood. As shall be demonstrated, this latter system of thought became the basis for Western ideas about health through the seminal work of Galen.

In all of the above-mentioned cultures it was thought that a person was in a state of health when all of the humors were in dynamic equilibrium. This equilibrium, however, was sensitive to the individual's age, sex, and temperament in relation to the climate in which the individual lived, the seasons, the specific food consumed, and other acts of daily living. An in-depth study of these multiple factors within a frame of reference of the individual as a whole formed the basis for the diagnosis. Treatment was oriented toward the modification of factors that might be disruptive of the harmonic functioning of the organism as a whole. Interestingly, all three of these systems—Chinese, Indian, and Mediterranean—became the authoritative avenues of scientific learning of their time within the same one-thousand-year period, from approximately the fifth century B.C. to the fifth century A.D.

The Universal Order

The most commonly known philosophy of the Chinese in regard to health is concisely stated in a very old Chinese proverb:

> The ancient sages did not treat those who were already ill; they instructed those who were not ill.

As an aside, this statement is, without doubt, the epitome of the emphasis in current holistic health practices on the importance of instructing well people in the appreciation of the practice and maintenance of high levels of wellness. The basis of this holistic health concept is embedded in a major tenet of Chinese philosophy that can trace its origins back in millennia of time. It is the conviction that man's nature is part of a universal order.[1]

The Macrocosm–Microcosm Paradigm

The logic of the Chinese philosophy runs something like this: it is because the universe is orderly that it is meaningful. Since the universe is meaningful, humans can derive the laws of nature under which the universe operates and thereby learn to predict its actions. A person as an intrinsic part of the universe is also of the nature of this universal order, and thus can know himself or herself by consistent, systematic investigation of self based upon principles that reflect the accepted model of the universe as macrocosm. In so regarding an individual as a microcosm of the universe, by inductive logic Chinese thought has developed extensive schemata to explain the multiple interconnections that are posited for this individual and universe relationship.

Phase Energetics

In regard to health, the macrocosm–microcosm paradigm suggests that there is a constant interaction and exchange of energies between the universe and each individual. Illness is thus seen as some kind of imbalance in the incessant and mutual flow between universe and individual. This flow is assessed within the local context of the natural meteorologic, climatologic, and immunologic modifications at a particular time, which is calculated according to the epicycles of solar and lunar energies. This concept, translated from the Chinese as "phase energetics," has its origins in the Taoist cosmology of about the eighth century A.D.;[2] however, the regular rhythms of natural events were noted in the most primitive times as well.

As was noted in Chapter 2, one of the first indications of man's appreciation of the ubiquity of rhythms in nature was reflected in the ancient fertility rituals that were performed according to various lunar cycles. Signatures of man's recognition of the cyclic passing of time dating back as far as 35,000 B.C. have been excavated by archeologists and these clearly indicate man's identification of the relationship of the lunar phases and solar cycles with food gathering.[3] Called *cupules*, these indicators were made of stones that had been shaped circularly, each with a hole through the center and with smaller depressions or pits around the periphery. Etched or scratched into the circular stones were figures of animals, their faces frequently oriented so that the pit in the stone became the eye of the animal. Sometimes these forms were accompanied by outlines of plants. By directing the cupule toward the north at night, the shadow cast by the moon over the lip of the pit onto the figures of the animals or plants would indicate the phases of the moon, and the angle of the shadows would mark the time of the year (the season). Engmann suggests that in this way the time of migrations of certain animals and the ripening of particular edible plants were determined by the ancients of the Neolithic period.

Both the hieroglyphics of the ancient Egyptians and the ideograms of the ancient Chinese speak with respect for the natural cycles of sun, moon, stars, and seasons. The recurrence of the latter provided a basis for the underlying philosophy of eternal life which pervaded both of these cultures. However, the unique addition that Chinese thought appended to these ideas was the concept of simultaneity; that is, that there could be a logical connection between two effective events, both of which exist in the same time but in different places in space. This concept of synchroneity is in direct contradistinction to the logic of causality which became dominant in the more recent Western view of health and illness.

The Five Evolutive Phases

The ideas on phase energetics began to be systematized by Tsou Yen, who is thought to have lived between approximately 350 to 270 B.C. Five major energetic qualities, the individual physical processes, distinguished the macrocosmic influences on the microcosm. These qualities, called then (as now) wood, fire, earth, metal, and water, are seemingly related in sequence, and their powers or dominances over one another are also related sequentially. Because of this natural cycling in time, they have been translated from the Chinese as the "Five Evolutive Phases."

Orbisiconography

The development of information on the macrocosmic–microcosmic energetic interchange for the individual is exceedingly detailed, systematic, and comprehensive. The basis of this interchange concerns a spectrum or "orb" of functions and relationships of body parts to their physiology. For this reason Porkert and others have agreed to call its study *orbisiconography* (*tsang-hsiang*). The case history within this system would include information on whether the orb of the person who is being diagnosed is *yin* or *yang*, and the particular subsystem it is in (*e.g., yin* in *yin, yin* in *yang, etc.*). The Five Evolutive Phases are analyzed to determine the cyclic position of the orb. It is also determined whether the orb is male or female and what its essential energetic nature is. Its quality and the effects that would be in opposition or injurious to that quality are also determined. The energetic patterning of the individual, his or her sound, the vocal expression of emotions or feelings that are involved with the illness, and the characteristic coloring of the person are all detailed. Because different foods contain different combinations of *yin–yang* patterning, corresponding cereals, domestic animals, and the class of animals are also included in the description of the orb for information to be used both symbolically and for the nutritional planning for the individual. In determining how the orb of the individual is intersecting with the macrocosm, several other factors are taken into consideration. Prime among these is the hour of the day as indicated by the positions of the sun and the moon. Relationships are then determined in reference to a particular planet, to the seasons, and to both universal and terrestrial time.

The next consideration is the interconnection of the orb with the microcosm, that is, with the individual. The relationship with the orb of a complementary polarity is decided upon, and consideration is given to the counteraction of the effects of the next orb in sequence. The radial pulse (there are twelve pulses, three that are superficial and three that are felt more deeply in the tissues at each wrist) of concern is specified. Also, the relevant sinarteries, or meridians (conduits of energy concerned with the processing, storage, and distribution of ch'i, the life energy), are mapped.

Important to the diagnosis is how the orb feels. Consequently there is an inspection of specific areas on the body's surface, particular body openings, and sense organs to ascertain the response of the orb in the physical body. Attention is given to the psychic reactions or emotions involved with the condition and any secretion of fluid which may accompany that reaction. The bearing and outward behavior of the individual are taken into account, and dream motifs of the individual are analyzed for further information to check which orb it is that is disturbed.

Finally, the specific and the dominant functions of the orb are assessed; the manner in which the orb acts, the way the physiologic energy is contained within the individual, and other characteristics and functions of the orb are delineated in detail.[1]

Basic Ancient Chinese Literature

The literature on which this information profile is based is quite old. The major reference, *The Yellow Emperor's Classic of Internal Medicine*, was written about 200 B.C. It contains information on anatomy and physiology which is not similar to Western concepts. Included also is information on hygiene, acupuncture, and moxibustion. The two last are modes stimulating the flow of ch'i, in the former case by the insertion and twirling of sharp-pointed thin needles into the acupoints, and in the latter case by the concentrated use of heat over the acupoints.

The Materia Medica of Shen-nung, another classic, was written before 220 A.D. It describes 365 drugs divided into three categories according to (1) those which nourish life, (2) those which nourish nature, and (3) those which cure disease.

Another unusual book that is regarded as a standard reference is titled *Important Prescriptions Worth Treasuring in the Golden Chamber*. This was written in 200 A.D. by Chang Chung-ching. This work classifies diseases according to their major symptoms. The treatise contains 262 prescriptions, many of which continue to be used effectively by contemporary health practitioners.

The Concept of Simultaneity

The Chinese view was focused primarily on how humans function in relation to the rhythms of the universe. Over the centuries, Chinese influence spread far beyond the borders of ancient Cathay. Unlike

Western concepts of cure based on causal theories and analysis, the Chinese rationale was based on a concept of simultaneity; that is, that related events can occur synchronously although they may not occupy the same space. In this we see that the Chinese thought of time as well as space as being multidimensional.

Diagnostic Methods

Unlike the developments in the West, the Chinese did not develop an organic view of anatomy, nor did they consider sciences such as histology and biochemistry of primary importance. Their alternative view was supported by applied theories on orbisiconography (functional relationships within the body), sinarteriology (the natural channeling of the *ch'i* energy through conduits in the individual, which are called *meridians*), pharmacodynamics, climatology, and immunology.

Within this schema there are four diagnostic methods that are relevant: (1) inspection or examination of selected regions of the body and body orifices, (2) an extensive case history which is obtained directly from the patient, (3) the touching and smelling of different body parts, and (4) the auditory response to auscultation over body cavities. This methodologic approach was most effective for the early treatment of symptoms (in persons in whom the illness had not progressed to organic change) and for the early diagnosis and prevention of organic disease. Cardiac failure, diabetes, and cancer might fall into this latter category.

Another area of expertise is of interest because it clearly demonstrates the contrary perceptions of Chinese and Western medicine. For instance, periodic outbreaks of illness in large populations are perceived in the Chinese model as being due to a lack of specific energies in certain orbs at a particular solar–lunar time. This lack makes the resistance to disease difficult. In the interpretation of Western medicine, the same illness would be labeled as being due to a virus. Sometimes because the microbial base is indistinct, the diagnosis would be tentative, but nevertheless it would have a "name" which would seemingly remove the mystery.

Yin–Yang as Poles of a Continuum

Sensitivity to early symptoms, and therefore the facility with preventive measures, is based on the Chinese perception that change does not occur suddenly but rather that conversion from one state to another takes place gradually and in an unbroken progression along a continuum. The poles of this continuum are conditions of *yin* at one extremity and conditions of *yang* at the other. The concept of *yin–yang* is not one of dichotomous entities because each polarity contains within itself a seed of its opposite (note the representation of these seeds by the light and dark circles within *yin* and *yang* in Fig. 3–1). Consequently, there is a smooth and natural progression in the *yin–yang* continuum from, for instance, conditions of *yin* in *yin* ➭ *yang* in *yin* ➭ *yang* in *yang* ➭ *yin* in *yang* ➭ *yin* in *yin,* and so on. This progression is constantly shifting in sequence through solar–lunar time and therefore the cosmic energies that play upon the microcosm, the individual, are also in constant flux. In modern terminology we would call these energies *exogenous biorhythms,* biorhythms that are caused by external sources such as the sun and the moon. One category of these biorhythms is concerned with the circadian rhythms (*e.g.,* sleep–wake cycles), which are regulated by the dark–light periods of the day.

The *yin–yang* theory of polarity has appeared in the literature since the fourth century B.C., but apparently the concept was known for as much as a thousand years before that.[5] Sinologists note that *yin* and *yang* are generic terms for the polar aspects of effects, and as such they are not directly translatable into many languages other than Chinese. Over the two to three thousand years during which the idea of the *yin–yang* polarity has been known, many connotations have been assigned to it. Porkert has done an exhaustive technical analysis of these associations based upon *The Inner Classic of the Yellow Sovereign.*[6] By synthesizing his translations of these myriad associations, one can appreciate the fullness of the *yin–yang* polarity within a modern perspective.

In general, Porkert assigns the active aspect of an effective position to *yang,* which he designates as *actio,* from the Latin meaning an effect that takes place outside or beyond the position under consideration. For *yin,* the term *structive* is assigned, which is derived from the Latin *struere,* to form concretely, to construct. For example, within Porkert's framework a stimulus is *actio* (*yang*), whereas a response would be *structive* (*yin*). The logic follows directly, for just as it is only through the response that the stimulus can be perceived, so also the *yang* energies are made manifest in the *yin.* It would seem that perhaps *yang* could refer to the contemporary term, force field, and *yin* could be perceived as the test object of the field energies.

It is stated that *yang* refers to events that are not readily experienced and, therefore, are beyond empirical definition. *Yang* as process initiates several states: it is "something" setting loose, "something" transforming, "something" beginning, "something" dynamizing, developing, expanding, growing. It is "something" which cancels, annihilates, or is burned up (entropy?). *Yang* is "something" indeterminate yet determining, beyond direct experience yet capable of being perceived indirectly. Finally, *yang* is capable of fulfilling potentiality, but it cannot go beyond inherent tendencies.

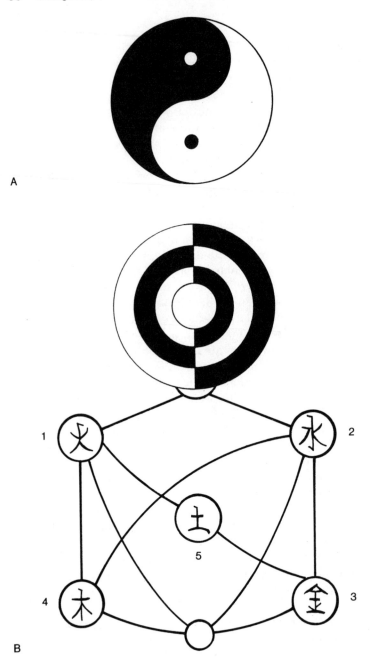

A

B

Fig. 3–1.
A illustrates the incessant intertwining of *yin* (dark) and *yang* (light) polarities, and that within the *yin* is the *yang* representation (*light circle*) and within the *yang* the *yin* representation (*dark circle*). B is a copy of an old Taoist drawing showing the interconnections between the *yin–yang* and the Five Evolutive Phases: *1* equals fire, *2* equals water, *3* equals metal, *4* equals wood, and *5* equals earth. *(Redrawn from Paols S: The Chinese Art of Healing. New York, Herder & Herder, 1971)*

Yin, on the other hand, is concerned with "something" finished or completed which had been actively (*yang*) initiated. It is therefore "something" confirming, responsive. It is "something" reposing, quiescent, static, and "something" substantive, consolidating, and becoming perceptible. It is "something" becoming rigid, dying off, or fading away, yet "something" preserving and conserving. *Yin* has a tendency to transform a transient effect into a lasting one, to preserve evanescent qualities. It is "something" condensing or concentrating, closing in. *Yin* suggests "something" awaiting organization, yet "something" determinate. Porkert notes that the use of *yin* and *yang* as qualifiers always calls to mind *all* of the fundamental associations. Consequently, the use of *yin–yang* within this context of definitions speaks to many dimensions at once and so gives voice to the underlying sense of simultaneity that was noted above as being a distinctive characteristic of the Chinese view of health. This grasp of constant change is impressive, particularly when one remembers that to the *yin–yang* polarity is added the qualitative cyclic factors of the Five Evolutive Phases, the energetic qualities that constantly change over the course of time (Table 3–1).

Associations Beyond *Yin–Yang* and the Five Evolutive Phases

Associations between *yin* and *yang* and the Five Evolutive Phases shown in Table 3–1 are ascertainable in the actual practice of acupuncture. There are also two nonobservable factors (that is, the specific energies can be ascertained, but they do not have underlying physical organs), both of which relate to the fire phase of the Five Evolutive Phases. These are the *pericardium* (*yin*), which should not be mistaken for the cardiac pericardium as it is known in Western anatomy, and a meridian, or sinartery, called the *Tri-warmer* (*yang*).

Discussing the efficacy of these concepts of phase energetics, a recent Department of Health, Education and Welfare publication states the following:

Primitive as it may sound, the concept (of phase energetics)

Table 3–1.
Associations Between *Yin* and *Yang* and the Five Evolutive Phases

Evolutive Phase		Yin	Yang
Wood	corresponds to the	Liver	Gallbladder
Fire	corresponds to the	Heart	Small intestines
Earth	corresponds to the	Spleen	Stomach
Metal	corresponds to the	Lungs	Large intestines
Water	corresponds to the	Kidneys	Urinary bladder

properly applied by experienced acupuncturists has been achieving seemingly remarkable medical results as witnessed most recently by United States visitors to the People's Republic of China.[7]

Categories of Pathogenesis

Yin and *yang* are but forms of *ch'i*, a generic term for universal life energy. All diseases are considered to be due to congestion or stasis of this free-flowing energy. In all there are three categories of pathogenesis:

1. Where the causes are intrinsic to the individual (the contemporary category here would be psychosomatic illness). The Chinese have related seven distinct emotions to this division; joy (which has only recently been recognized in Western crisis theory to be a causative factor in illness), anger, sorrow, worry, grief, fear, and terror.

2. Where the causes are extrinsic or external to the individual. Six climatic conditions come under this rubric: cold, warmth, dryness, wetness, wind, and heat.

3. Finally, there are those illnesses which individuals bring upon themselves through "unnatural acts," such as eating an inadequate diet, or emotional excesses.

Ch'i, the Universal Life Energy

Ch'i is both patterned and specific. There is *ch'i* as the vital potential inborn in each person which maintains that person until death. There is an aspect of *ch'i* that is both defensive and compensatory and that maintains physiologic harmony. There is primordial *ch'i* related to the earth energy, magnetism. There is also a distinctive *ch'i* energy that confines itself to the *yang* hours of the day as well as a *ch'i* energy that finds expression during the *yin* hours.

Conditions of *Ch'i*

Porkert lists 32 conditions of *ch'i* pertinent to health in humans.[8] Among the more important are those *ch'i* energies that affect the individual in cycles 2 weeks apart, those that are responsible for the momentary condition of the body, and the *ch'i* energy that moves in the sinarteries (meridians) and is used in acupuncture and moxibustion. There is *ch'i* as free or potential energy, *ch'i* concerned with macrocosmic influences, constructive *ch'i* energy, *ch'i* energy that opposes the normal circulation with pathologic consequences, *ch'i* concerned with the immunology of the body, and *ch'i* energy that is assimilated from food. Rhythmic energies concerned with respiration are vital to life, as are all *yin–yang* physiologic energies. There is energy that results from a synthesis of cosmic and individual energies, the cosmic energy that the individual assimilates by breathing, and true *ch'i* that sustains the integrity of the individual and defends the individual against disturbances of his or her dynamic equilibrium.

Over the millennia of Chinese thought on human energetics, particular attention has been paid to those phenomena that occur regularly and without variance. From this rich lode of observation a vast but thorough documentation of qualitatively different aspects of human energy forms has been assembled so that the term *ch'i* always refers to energy of a specific and definable quality. This means that *ch'i* always refers to distinctive and identifiable qualitative patterns of energy, although when used by itself, the term *ch'i* also may be used in a generic sense.

Forms of *Ch'i* Crucial to Human Health

The literature, particularly *The Inner Classic of the Yellow Sovereign*, is replete with categorizations of the forms by which *ch'i* manifests in the human body. The following resumé is of some of the forms of energy that are most crucial to the valid understanding of health within the Chinese perspective.

Ching is a fundamental form of energy that cannot be directly perceived by the five physical senses but, nevertheless, is a prerequisite or substratum for life. Definite polarity becomes apparent, although the energy still cannot be directly perceived, with *shen*. *Shen* is invested with a definite organizing and transforming quality that molds the individual's character and maintains it. In an attempt to define *shen* in contemporary terms, one might conceive it as the nexus where field forces involved with the shaping of the human organism and the biochemical elements that are mediated through the physiologic functions of the pregnant mother meet.

Directly related to *ching* and *shen*, and as aspects of them, are the energetic forces *p'o* and *hun*. In reference to *yin–yang*, Porkert quotes an ancient commentary that states that "... *shen* corresponds to *yang* in *yang*, and *p'o* to *yang* in *yin*."[9] In contemporary terms, it would seem that from *hun* derive the forces that actively mold the personality of the person, and from *p'o* comes the anchoring of psychic functions in the individual.

Hsüeh is a vital fluid the source of which is the energy of food. *Hsüeh* is the receptacle, or *yin* aspect, of *ch'i*. It is said that when the two, *ch'i* and *hsüeh*, are in harmony the vital energies flow in the meridians and ". . . an individual may be constituted." In contemporary terms, it would seem that this refers to the quickening of the fetus which occurs at about 3 months after conception.

There is a complementarity between *hsuëh* and another form of energy, *mo*, and they are considered polar opposites. *Mo* is governed by time and in one sense may be considered to be the pulse by which *hsuëh* is contained and circulated throughout the body. The timing of the *mo* appears to be directly related to the body's metabolic rhythms. Moving within the conduits (meridians or sinarteries) is *ying*, an energetic form basic to metabolism. Its complement, *wei*, moves outside the conduits and is concerned with the defenses of the body. *Wei* is also responsible for the healthy condition of the body as seen in the warmth of the flesh, the coloring of the complexion, the openness of the pores of the skin, the sheen of the hair, the mobility of the joints, and the ability of the body to defend itself against pathogenic intrusion. Another form of energy, which is also written as *wei* in English translations but not so in the original Chinese characters, refers to the distinctive taste of flavor of food or drugs that figure importantly in the pharmacodynamics of the Chinese.

Two complementary body fluids, *chin* and *yeh*, also form a polarity. *Chin* seems to be concerned with waste products, such as sweat, and may be involved in temperature regulation through perspiration. *Yeh* results from the assimilation of food. This body fluid "irrigates the bones," fortifies the energy of the brain and the medulla oblongata, and gives a healthy glow to the complexion.

Hsing is a form of energy which gives definite structure and proportion to the physical body and corresponds to body muscles and flesh. Out of the Taoist alchemic tradition comes the concept of *ling*, a form of energy which impresses on the body the marks of energetic influences to which the body has been exposed.

Sinarteries and Acupoints

Based upon the extensive conception of phase energetics, the Chinese developed a most distinctive and unique contribution to world thought, a systematic theory of conduits of energy (sinarteries) and sensitive points on them (acupoints) which underlie the health and vigor of the body. This theory is essential to the understanding of Chinese diagnosis, pharmacotherapy, and massage, and it is the theoretical foundation of both acupuncture and moxibustion. Porkert notes that it is the sensitive points, the discovery of which was probably based on the symptoms that accompanied illness, that provide the observable and primary data on which the theory is based. These sensitive points can be demonstrated under controlled laboratory conditions with modern research apparatus to measure the electrical resistance or thermosensitivity of the skin. On the other hand, these sinarteries continue to be rationally explained on the basis of systematic speculations, for there is no anatomic substratum posited for them. Conceptually they seem to be analogous to lines of force in, for instance, a magnetic field. These lines of force form a network for the energetic flow of the body.

Acupuncture and Moxa Treatment

The purpose of acupuncture or moxibustion at the sensitive points on the skin surface is to restore the energy flow of the body to its proper rhythm or cycling. These sensitive points are thoroughly and precisely mapped. When they are stimulated, either by piercing the skin with thin needles in acupuncture or by the application of the burning ash of moxa, the mugwort plant (*Artemisia vulgaris*), to the acupoints, specific body reactions are thought to occur. Acupuncture and moxa treatment are sometimes combined.

Acupuncture is based on an analysis of the state of *ch'i*, as noted above. Acupuncture, being part of a holistic view, is not generally used by itself, but rather in conjunction with herbs and other medications, massage, breathing disciplines, and body work such as *T'ai-chi ch'uan*, a martial art.

I Ching: Sourcebook on Predictable Cyclic Behavior

Another ancient Chinese source of information to which the individual has resource in order to gain insight into the constant interplay of dynamic forces at the various levels of human organization is the *I Ching*, or *Book of Changes*. The *I Ching* is over 2000 years old and is used as a tool for learning about one's self and also as a method of divination, of getting information on future events.

The name of the book itself, *The Book of Changes*, epitomizes the philosophy that is stated above. In ancient Chinese thought there was only *Tai Ch'i*, the Absolute, the Macrocosm. However, *Tai Ch'i* is known by the observable behaviors that at the microcosmic level are seen as constant movement or change, for no situation remains the same from one moment to another. This continual flux proceeds in predictable cyclic routines in accordance with universal and observable laws that are based upon the interaction of *yin* and *yang*.

The cyclic *yin–yang* interactions concern every event in nature, so that there is a universal net of connectives binding all matter, animate and inanimate, in space and time. In this manner each event or behavior of an individual is intrinsically related to the whole of things, to the entire universal state of affairs then prevailing, that is, the current change. Since all cyclic phenomena are predictable, it is possible to foretell the shape of changes to come, and to interpret how the individual person's situation fits into the multitudinous interacting cycles. With this foreknowledge, the individual can proceed consciously and harmoniously with it. The procedure for consulting the *I Ching* (pronounced *ee djing*) depends primarily on the attitude with which one approaches the *I Ching*: it is to be approached as one would approach a wise sage. A question is framed in terms of the relationship between the specific moment and the future. For instance, one may ask "What is the meaning of _____?" or "How shall I plan for _____?" or "How will _____ develop itself in the future?"

A convention has been determined for the assignment of *yin* or *yang* to either the heads or tails of coins (three are used at once for a series of six throws) or a bunch of yarrow sticks (which are 50 in number although only 49 sticks will be used in the procedure). The coins or the yarrow sticks are tossed and the moment of the throw is considered to be an establishment of a relationship with relevant universal forces. The view is that every event (*i.e.*, the throwing of the coins or sticks) is but a part of a total simultaneous situation. The separation of the event from other events is only apparent, not real; that is, the event is a unified process in which separation seems real only from a limited perspective.

In the case of the coins, all three coins are thrown at the same time. Since each of the coins has two sides, there are 2^3 or 8 possible configurations in which the coins can land. Throwing the three coins three times in succession gives one a trigram. Each pattern of the final positions of the three coins gives one either a *yin* line, a *yang* line, or a changing *yin* or *yang* line in the trigram. The first trigram constitutes the lower trigram, and the process is repeated to obtain the upper trigram. Together the lower and upper trigrams constitute a hexagram. In the case in which any of the lines are a changing *yin* or a changing *yang*, another hexagram is thrown. The second hexagram is indicative of what will happen after the conditions of the first hexagram are met. Once one has obtained a hexagram, the *I Ching* may be consulted. There are oracles for 64 hexagrams. Since any of the lines of a hexagram can change and give rise to another hexagram, there are 64^2 or 4,096 possible answers to questions.

The advice in *I Ching* is given in metaphors, and therefore analogy is used to interpret the divinations. Since the divination is for the individual alone, the symbolism in which the answer is cloaked has a deeply personal meaning to that individual.[10] By this self-referential system the individual gains an understanding of the ordering principles of his or her daily life.

Shamanic Mode of Divination Similar to *I Ching*—the *Fa*

It is of considerable interest to note that there is a shamanic mode of divination in Dahomey, Africa similar to *I Ching*. To see the future and therefore to know with certainty how to act, one visits a person who knows how to "draw the *Fa*." The *Fa* has a threefold nature:

1. The *Fa* is the greatest god.
2. The *Fa* is the father of 1000 *voodoo* demons.
3. The *Fa* is regarded as the personal genie of the person who is consulting him.

The method of drawing the *Fa* is as follows. A string of date pits is thrown once the question is asked. The pits fall either concave side up or convex side up. Each position of the date pits is related to a numeral that is then referred to in a reference table that gives the hierarchial order of the prevailing demons. This exposes the minor demons who are involved.

Each of the demons is connected with a particular myth. The real situation can be determined by analogy from the myth. The deciphering of the metaphors is said to create a particular state of mind in the person consulting the *Fa* and the person can then take action. The validity of the oracle is proved by the effectiveness of the consulter's action.

Due largely to Jungian interpretations of the symbolic relationship between the inquirer and the *I Ching,* there has been a recent resurgence of interest in this *Book of Changes*. However, the reason why it is effective is not known. To find an appropriate answer perhaps one must once again go back 2,000 years, again to the Chinese:

> He who knows does not speak,
> He who speaks does not know.
> Lao Tse

Summary

As can be seen from the preceding pages, Chinese thoughts on health appear to be the most whole of all holistic health perspectives. Within the Chinese paradigm the person as an individual is in direct confrontation with the potent forces of the known universe, and learns to live in harmony with them in a manner that is most constructive for his future well-being.

To understand this relationship between the individual and the universe, the individual is thrown back on his or her own hunches and intuitions, and this exploration of self provides a key to the dynamics of the unconscious. It is out of this active awareness of the unconscious life that the person begins to understand and take responsibility for self. This personal responsibility for self is also the goal of the contemporary holistic health movement, to which Chinese thought continues to be a major contributor.

The current interest in traditional Chinese health concepts, like the emergence of the present popular interest in holistic health practices, has been analyzed from many points of view. The consensus appears to be that the following have been the major stimuli for both:

1. The large incidence of harmful side-effects from synthetic drugs, and the publication of this information in the public media

2. The analytic nature of modern Western medicine, and the resultant large amount of specialization of physicians along with the concomitant decrease in regard for the understanding of the "whole person"

3. A general disregard of the patient's complaints and impressions about his or her own illness in favor of an emphasis on the causal aspects of disease[11]

Although the People's Republic of China has done away with much of the ancient traditions in a concentrated search to ameliorate the living conditions of a present population which approaches one billion people, the validity of the universal principle of *yin–yang* is still proclaimed in present-day China. Even the prestigious *Red Flag*, an official People's Republic of China periodical, stated that ". . . the law of the unity of opposites is the basic law of the universe."[12]

References

1. Topley M: Chinese traditional etiology. In Leslie C (ed): Asian Medical Systems, p 250. Berkeley, University of California Press, 1976
2. Porkert M: The Theoretical Foundations of Chinese Medicine, p 55. Cambridge, the Massachussetts Institute of Technology Press, 1974
3. Engmann RD: Introductory remarks to Session II. In Engmann RD (ed): Third Conference on Planetology and Space Mission Planning. Ann NY Acad Sci 187:125–130, 1972
4. Porkert, *op cit*, pp 113–114
5. Porkert, *op cit*, p 23
6. Porkert, *op cit*, pp 14–23
7. Chen JYP: Acupuncture. In Medicine and Public Health in the People's

Republic of China, p 68. Washington, DC, Department of Health, Education and Welfare, Publication #(NIH) 73–67, 1973

8. Porkert, *op cit*, pp 168–173
9. Porkert, *op cit*, p 184
10. Blofeld J (trans): I Ching: the Book of Changes, pp 59–71. New York, EP Dutton, 1968
11. Otanka Y: Chinese traditional medicine in Japan. In Leslie C (ed): Asian Medical Systems, p 322. Berkeley, University of California Press, 1976
12. Ch'in-wen H: Mao Tse-Tung thought lights up the way for advances of China's medical science. Selections From the Mainland Magazine #675–755:49–63, Hong Kong, the American Consulate General, 1970

4 The Indian Sphere of Influence

In order to understand the Indian influence on health practices, one must first understand the ancient philosophy of the Indian people, particularly the Hindus and the Buddhists. For both of these groups only the inward search was important; the concept of health developed within that context.

The *Rg-Veda*, the oldest literature of the Indian people, is considered to contain the highest truth; all else, it is said, is commentary. The word *veda* itself means wisdom or science. The *Rg-Veda* dates back to the latter part of the second millenium B.C. and consists of two parts: the *mantras* are the primary source, and the *Bramanas* are the illustrative commentaries. Included in the *Rg-Veda* are the *Upanishads*, which deal with broad philosophical problems.

An indicator of the perspective in which health was regarded is the term *bhisoj*. As used in the *Rg-Veda*, it means a healer of disease who is also conversant with healing herbs (*Rg-Veda:* x.97.6). Miraculous cures of blindness, lameness, and leprosy are frequently mentioned (*Rg-Veda:* 112, 116–117, 120, x.39–40, *etc.*). Soma, the divine king of plants, was considered to be a healing deity (*Rg-Veda:* vi.74). Transgressions, particularly of moral law, were thought to be punished with diseases.[1] The most frequent disease visited on individuals for this purpose seems to have been dropsy, an abnormal accumulation of fluid in the tissues and body cavities which is currently associated primarily with kidney or heart disease or with cirrhosis of the liver.

The Vedic View

The Vedic view is that there is nothing that is absolutely stable in the universe. Rather, all is in collective movement (*jigatī*). Nevertheless, this underlying motion has an intrinsic organization which demonstrates itself as order in the universe, and this order is meaningful. The order over vast periods of time is enduring and, therefore, this long duration makes it seem as though there is stability. The ceaseless movement is perceived by the senses and is experienced and thus known; however, this knowing is therefore at least twice removed from the actual reality. Because of this, the teachings hold that we can only know directly by removing our attention from the sensed or objective universe and exploring deeply our individual subjective nature.

The *Bhutas* and the *Pranas*

The living physical body is made up of dual qualities, the *bhutas*, which constitute the matter and the senses of the body, and the *prana*, the life energy that is vital and holds together the physical form as an organic whole. The former is made up of two classes of material, *parāmanus*, which are discrete factors that are made up of atomic particles that, however, have no magnitude and are to be considered something like mathematical points. Chatterji suggests that this is a state yet to be found by Western scientists[2]; however, one would suspect that *neutrinos*, which are particles that have no mass, charge, or magnetic properties but can pass through the matter of the whole earth, are good candidates. The second class of the *bhutas* is the *Ākasha*, or Continuum, which is made up of an infinite number of force field vectors and which fills all space.

The *paramānus* are related to what we in Western culture would call the four humors. These sensations are temperature (heat or cold), color, flavor, and odor, and are symbolically referred to as fire, earth, water, and air, respectively. The sensation of sound, however, derives from the *Ākasha*, or Continuum. This special placement of sound is owing to the fact that sound, unlike the four humors, does not need discrete forms of matter to be perceived (*i.e.*, through thermal agitation of atoms, or through photons, or by way of chemical compounds that travel through fluid for flavor and through air to convey odor). The freedom of sound from a material conveyor can be observed today in the use of the radio to communicate music and messages.

Avenues of Perception

The daily activities of living are carried out by the senses through two avenues of perception, the nervous system or cognitive senses and those senses functioning through the muscles, such as the sense of position in space that is based on proprioception, locomotion, and so on. There are also the analytic mental functions, the five senses, the ego-complex (the container of "various bits of experiences" upon which the sense of "I" is based), the conceptual field, the buddhic or intuitive functions that give us a sense of oneness or unity, and the *Atman* or Self.[3]

Yoga as a Basis
for Unitive Perception

Based upon this unitive understanding of the individual as a multifaceted being, but one who is rooted in the Real or the Absolute, Indian thought developed methods for the unfoldment of consciousness, which is collectively known as *yoga*. The fundamental purpose of all forms of yoga is to reach total enlightenment, *samādhi*. All efforts are directed toward its achievement (Table 4–1).

Yoga is practiced to speed up the natural evolution of the individual through the ignorance and suffering that are the conditions of life. The underlying philosophy is based on an unalterable determination to persevere, life after life, until the yogi is perfected physically, emotionally, mentally, and morally. Such, it is believed, will be the ultimate state of all life, but through yogic practices the yogi accelerates his or her individual progress.

In the course of practicing yogic techniques, psychic powers or *siddhis*—some of which are known today as extrasensory, higher sensory, or ultrasensory perceptions—are acquired as a natural by-product of the effort. In the process, the yogi gains a deeply personal knowledge of the nature of the mind and mental perception, of the nature of desire and its bonding effects, and, finally, of the nature of

Table 4–1.
Aspects of Yoga and Their Interrelationships

Aspects of Yoga	Area of Functional Mastery	Yogic Control
I. Hatha yoga	Breath	Physical body and vitality
II. Laya yoga	Will	Powers of mind
1. Bhakti yoga	Love	Powers of divine love
2. Shakti yoga	Energy	Energizing forces of nature
3. Mantra yoga	Sound	Powers of sound vibrations
4. Yantra yoga	Form	Powers of geometric form
III. Dhyāna yoga	Thought	Powers of thought processes
IV. Raja yoga	Method	Powers of discrimination
1. Jñāna yoga	Knowledge	Powers of intellect
2. Karma yoga	Activity	Powers of action
3. Kundalini yoga	Kundalini	Powers of psychic–nerve force
4. Samādhi yoga	Self	Powers of ecstasy

(Based on Evans-Wentz WY: Tibetan Yoga and Secret Doctrines, p 33. London, Oxford University Press, 1967)

liberation from the restrictions of the human condition and the results of that freedom.

The *Nadis* as Conduits of Human Energy

Very similar to the Chinese thought, there is a concept in Indian thought of nonobservable channels or conduits of energy that vitalize the physical body. However, these channels of force have no physical substratum. They are referred to as the *nadis*, from the Sanskrit *nad*, which means "movement." The number of these *nadis* is variously noted as being anything from 72,000 to 727,200,000; however, of this number only 14 *nadis* are recognized to be major. Three of the fourteen are considered to be the principle *nadis*, the *sushumna*, the *ida*, and the *pingala*, and they are described in considerable detail.[4]

Citta, the Basis for Sensory Input

There are three types of energies concerned with health: *prana*, the life energy underlying the organization of the life process; *kundalini*, which is concerned with creative energy in the sense approximated by the Western term *libido*; and, finally, there is an energy that is somewhat akin to the concept of *eros*, or love. Whatever state *prana* is in, it is in an energy-rich form in health.

As *prana* runs through the *nadis* it acts as a conveyor for *citta*, the psyche's willful, emotional, and intellective activities. It is *citta* that puts us in contact with the environment through sensory input. In one of the forms of yoga, *hatha* yoga, the aim is the conscious control of *citta*, so that it flares up as a fire (*hatha* means the violent arrest of the inconstancy and uncertainty of *citta*). When in control, illumination is released through the *sushumna*. The *citta* gradually becomes purified, and this leads to serenity (*samādhi*). *Sakti*, an active force, governs the process.

The Primary *Nadi*, *Sushumna*

The pranic currents move and circulate through the nadis in a manner that is related to the sun, the moon, and the condition of the individual. *Sushumna* is the principal *nadi*, and it is described as running up a lumen in the middle of the spinal cord "like a thread through the eye of a needle." This lumen is reported to be the remnant of the hollow tube from which the spinal cord and the brain developed embryologically.[4] It is described quite precisely as beginning 5 centimeters above the anus and 5 centimeters behind the penis and going to a nonobservable organ, called a *cakra*, a transducer of energies that enter the body. This particular *cakra* is situated in what we would call the biofield of the individual, with a physical locus between the eyebrows; it is called the *ajna cakra.*[5] The nature of the *cakras* will be discussed more fully below.

Ida and *Pingala,* the Lunar and Solar Energies

Ida and *pingala* start in the same place as the *sushumna.* Each goes around the spinal cord in serpentine fashion, but in opposite directions. *Ida* twines to the left; it is pale, lunar, and feminine. *Pingala* twists to the right; it is red, solar, and masculine. There is some suggestion that when the yogi is female the spiraling ascends in the direction opposite to that of the male yogi. *Ida* and *pingala* entwine as they ascend the spinal cord (actually the field counterpart of the spinal cord) and meet *sushumna* at the *ajna cakra* in a "triple knot." They then separate, the *ida* exiting through the left nostril and the *pingala* exiting through the right nostril.

The Arousal of *Kundalini*

These major nadis are stimulated when the energy *kundalini* is aroused from its latent state through controlled yogic practices. When *kundalini* is thus aroused it is said to be like a fire that burns everything impure in its path. Its goal is to reach two other *cakras,* one in the heart region and the other at the throat. This consuming fire or heat is obtained by the "transmutation" of sexual energies.[6]

Yoga is far removed from the ecstasy of shamanism. Its goal is *samādhi,* a state of the highest concentration, which comes only after the yogi has disciplined his or her fantasies, emotions, restless mind, and the physical body and its physiologic functioning. In *samādhi,* not only does the yogi have complete mastery of self, but in this state of consciousness the yogi also has a profound and personal experience of the sacred. In describing the great yogi Milarepa. Evans-Wentz states the process graphically: "As the chemist experiments with the elements of matter, Milarepa experimented with the elements of consciousness."[7]

The Concept of the *Cakras* as Transformers of Human Energy

The *raison d'etre* of yoga is the in-depth study of human consciousness. Unlike Western thought, which recognizes only the brain as the locus of human consciousness, Indian thought includes the concept of *cakras* which, as stated above, are physically nonobservable. They are described as patterned vortices of energy, the center of the vortex being connected with the *nadi sushumna* in the field counterpart of the lumen of the spinal cord. These vortices act as centers of consciousness for such awarenesses as space-consciousness, inner movement, emotion, and other qualitative expressions of the psyche.[8]

Through concentration and meditation, the practitioner activates the *cakras* and makes them more responsive to various levels of organization of the human energy systems. Polar forces come into play through the solar energies of *pingala*, which results in consciousness, and the lunar energies of *ida*, which is concerned with the subconscious or depth psychology of the individual. Basically, the yogi is involved in the task of integrating *ida* and *pingala*. However, that is to state the task too simply. In fact, the yogi seeks an actual transformation of consciousness rather than simple consciousness raising.

It is difficult to understand yogic practices except through the personal practice of them. The bases of the body of theory from which yogic practices derive are so unlike Western empiricism that the alternative most frequently is to accept them on the basis of faith—and the fundamental tenets of yoga clearly state that it is not enough for one to believe, one must know! Nevertheless, given this recognition, let us look at what is said about the seven major *cakras*.[9]

The Seven Major *Cakras*

In reference to the physical body, the lowermost *cakra*, the *mūlādhāra* (*mūla* = root), is located at the base of the spinal column between the anal orifice and the genital organs, the site of the sacrococcygeal plexus. It is here that *kundalini* "sleeps" in a latent state in such a position as to block access to the prime *nadi, sushumna*. It is said to be related to forces deep within the earth, to the cohesive power of matter, to inertia, the sense of smell, and so forth. It is the basis for the present evolutionary thrust on Earth.[10,11]

There is a spleen *cakra* that is concerned with the specialization, subdivision, and distribution of vitality that comes from the sun. From a Western physiologic point of view, the spleen is concerned with the regeneration of red blood cells. Red blood cells contain the porphyrin hemoglobin, a respiratory pigment that makes the cells (and therefore the blood) red. It is the function of hemoglobin to distribute oxygen to the tissues, a necessity since human metabolism is mainly oxidative. Biochemically, the hemoglobin molecule and the chlorophyll molecule (which accepts photons from the sun to initiate photosynthesis) are both tetrapyrroles, both porphyrins, and are very similar stereochemically. Therefore, the functions assigned to the spleen *cakra* seem rational from a Western point of view.

The *manipura cakra*, which is also called *nabhisthana* (*nabhi* = umbilicus), is situated in the lumbar region at the level of the umbilicus. It is related to the element fire, to the sun, to the menstrual flow, to breath, to the sense of sight, and to the transmission of organic substances into the psychic energies of the lower, more sensuous, emotions. From a current psychosomatic medical point of view, it is located in the area in which one gets peptic ulcers or "stomachaches" as a result of pent-up anger, anxiety, or other such emotional states.

The *anāhata* is the heart *cakra*, which is in the region of the heart. It is the seat of *prana*, the life energy, and of the *jivātman*, the individual soul. It is related to the element air, to the sense of touch, to the motor force, and to the blood system. In Western terms it regulates respiration, the heart, and the blood through the sympathetic nervous system. The *anāhata* governs the plane of human realization. One is reminded of the central principle of the Christ figure—that of love as the basis for the fulfillment of human life.

The *vishuddha cakra* is at the laryngeal and pharyngeal plexus, at the junction of the spinal column and the medulla oblongata. It is the seat of *udāna*, one of the five fires of sacrifice, and of the breath that carries the soul to the head in the *samādhi* state, the site of conscious transformation of *prana* through mantric power, the power of controlled sound. It is related to the *Akasha* (the Continuum), to the substrate of sound, and also to the skin.

The *ajna* (*ajna* = order, command) *cakra* is between the eyebrows, in the cavernous plexus. It is the seat of cognitive and subtle senses.

The *sahasrara*, also called the *brahmarandhra*, at the crown of the head, is represented by a thousand-petaled lotus (*sahasrā* = thousand). It is associated with the pituitary–pineal axis, and it is concerned with volition, acts of will, and altruism.

The Relationship Between the *Cakras* and the Five Elements

There is a relationship between the *cakras* and the five elements—earth, water, fire, air, and *akasha*—which is drawn upon in Ayurvedic health practices. For the yogi the understanding of this relationship rests on the knowledge of the Path of the Five Wisdoms, as personified by the Five Dhyāni Buddhas.[12] This knowledge is the essence of yogic teaching. In Western terms the Dhyāni Buddhas are analogous to the concept of universal force fields, the Thatness. *Vairochana* (which means "in shapes making visible") is the chief of the Dhyāni Buddhas and his region is the Central Realm. *Vairochana* is the source or manifestor of all phenomena. The Dhyāni Buddhas, therefore, symbolize those behaviors by which the yogi activates the *cakras*.

The *mūlādhāra* (root) *cakra* is related to the element earth, and its field of influence is concerned with ripening karma, rigidity, and routine activity. Its negative aspect is felt in the emotional energies of hatred. This *cakra* is symbolized by a cube (Fig. 4-1). The *manipura* (umbilicus or solar plexus) *cakra* is related to the element water. It represents a stage of assimilation of knowledges about the fundamental unity of all beings. Its full activation occurs where all self-limitation is

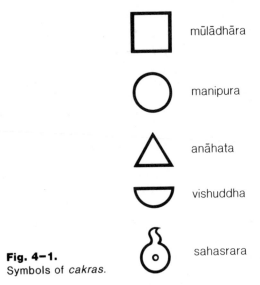

Fig. 4-1.
Symbols of *cakras*.

extinguished, where there is no longer a sense of duality between self and non-self. Its negative energies are fed by ego-conceit. The *manipura cakra* is symbolized by a sphere (Fig. 4-1).

The *anāhata* (heart) *cakra* is related to the element of fire and is symbolized by a cone or pyramid (Fig. 4-1). The sacrificial and compassionate nature of its energies transforms the personality and integrates its various aspects. The negative energy in this realm is envy.

The *vishuddha* (throat) *cakra* is related to the element air, and it is represented by a drawn bow (Fig. 4-1). This *cakra* is concerned with breath control and the use of vibratory sound, as in mantras. Its control manifests as discrimination and its negative energies are involved with passionate craving.

Finally, the *sahasrara* (crown) *cakra* is related to *Akasha*, the Continuum or element space. It is symbolized by a blue dot or flame (Fig. 4-1). It is considered a vehicle for the embodiment of universal law. Its negative aspects are involved with the fantasies and illusions of the *devas*, or angels. (See Fig. 4-2 for further commentary on the use of these symbols in mandalas and religious representations.)

The Universal Law of Karma

This complex conscious effort to attain fulfillment of being is complicated by the limitations of the human condition in which one finds one's self. These limitations are impersonally delineated by the natural and universal laws of karma; however, a unique ability of

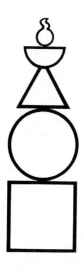

Fig. 4–2.
It is said that the body itself becomes a mandala during meditation, the visible becoming a symbol of a deeper reality. The remembrance of the *cakras* through their symbolic representations is built into the standard form of Indian *stupas* and Tibetan *chortens*, religious monuments or structures that were placed on the roads in those countries. Although the architecture differed, this line drawing is a basic representation of the fundamental model. The foundation is a cube which represents the root *cakra*, and the second story is a sphere representative of the solar plexus *cakra*. The middle story depicts the heart *cakra* by a triangle or pyramid. In the fourth story the throat *cakra* is symbolized by a semicircular bow, and the highest story is representative of the crown *cakra* which is symbolized by a flaming drop, the symbol of space. *(Based upon Govinda LA: Foundations of Tibetan Mysticism. London, Rider, 1969)*

human beings is the capacity for overcoming their conditions of life and passing beyond the delimitations.[13]

The laws of karma (action, work, destiny, product, and effect) are most fully developed within the Buddhist philosophy. The underlying base of this philosophy is that humans are an intrinsic part of a natural order governed by moral law. When an individual lives in accordance with these laws, there is opportunity to fully work through the conditions or experiences that life presents, and thus the individual dies having satisfied his or her *dharma,* or duty. However, if these conditions are evaded and life is not lived in accord with the natural order of the universe, the individual works against the energy bound up in these laws of interaction. Suffering results from this ignorance and further limiting conditions amass. It is then necessary for that individual to be born or reincarnated in order to learn the lessons of working in harmony with the natural law which he or she had not yet comprehended.[14]

The Tibetan Book of the Dead

These essentially Buddhist views on karma and rebirth are a logical outgrowth of a concept of life as a continuum of consciousness, in which death is but a serially recurring phase of successive lifetimes. The original transcripts of the Gautama Buddha's teachings were apparently destroyed over time in India (Buddha's birth occurred around the year 500 B.C.) and therefore the most authentic replications are those that were carried from India to Tibet and China.

The Tibetan Book of the Dead, the classic of Tibetan literature, was written in its current form in the eighth century A.D. as a text for

Mahayana Buddhism.[15] It may be read from two different perspectives: it contains instructions for the dying person that prepare the person for after-death experiences in *Bardo,* the realm of consciousness beyond physical existence; and it is also a text for serious students of yoga or other forms of learning about the psychic experiences of one's inner life. It is a profound book on the psychology of the human mind, teaching that in death as in life one becomes one's own judge. One of the verses tells of the potency of the image-making tendencies of the mind:

> O nobly born, whatever fearful or
> terrifying visions thou mayest see,
> recognize them to be but thine own
> thought forms.

The verse goes on to indicate that if the individual can remember this, the insight gained will help to release him or her from the power of those visions.[16]

The Tibetan Book of the Dead describes the psychic occurrences at the time of death so that the person will be prepared and will not enter that state in fear. It also gives an account of the dreamlike state one enters into immediately following death, and states specific instructions on how to conduct one's self while in *Bardo* and how to prepare for rebirth, describing prenatal events in some detail.

This knowledge is considered so important that, should a person not have access to it during his or her lifetime, it is recited at the deathbed either by the dying person or a monk or lama, for the major teaching is that the self of the dying or dead person is reflected in the godhead and dwells within. The understanding of this is crucial to the recognition that delimitations are self-induced and, therefore, that it is up to each individual to take responsibility for self. This principle of responsibility for self is a cornerstone for current holistic health practices.

The reason for reading *The Tibetan Book of the Dead* at the deathbed is that it cannot be assumed that the individual has this important knowledge. It is therefore considered a matter of high priority to bring this knowledge to the attention of all dying people. The psychologist Jung would agree with this point of view, for he says:

> It is a primordial, universal idea that the dead simply continue
> their earthly existence and do not know that they are disembodied
> spirits.[17]

Indian Knowledge
Based on Practical Experimentation

In addition to these personal knowledges based upon subjective experience, the people of ancient India had an advanced knowledge of chemicals based upon practical experimentation in the development of the arts of dye-making, tanning, soap-making, and the manufacture of glass and cement. Their understanding of herbs and roots is evidenced by the fairly recent introduction of one of them, *Rauwolfia*, into Western medicine, which opened up the whole field of tranquilizers and enlarged the spectrum of hypotensive drugs.

The historians Will and Ariel Durant write that even before the sixth century B.C. Hindu physicians described in remarkably accurate detail the ligaments, lymphatics, nerve facia, adipose and vascular tissues, and mucous and synovial membranes. These physicians had a thorough knowledge of digestive processes, including the various functions of gastric juices and the conversion of chyle into blood. The Code of Manu instituted many epidemiologic controls that cautioned against both the close association with or marriage to persons affected with tuberculosis, epilepsy, leprosy, chronic dyspnea, piles, and so forth. As early as 500 B.C. the Hindu medical schools were teaching birth control based on a rhythm method.

Fetal development was described accurately and in detail. For instance, it was noted that the sex of the fetus is not determinable for a period of time, and that under certain circumstances the growing embryo's sex could be influenced by food or drugs. In summing up this heritage of India, the Durants state that many Ayurvedic diagnoses and cures ". . . are still used in India with a success that is sometimes the envy of Western physicians."[18]

Ayurvedic Health Practices

Ayurveda translates as "the knowledge of life or longevity." *Ayur* implies that the concern is not limited to the curing of disease, but to the promotion of positive and vital health and longevity. The stated goal is "to cure the disease, to protect the healthy, and to prolong life" (Susruta: i.l.l and also Caraka: vi.1.4). The term *Veda* relates to the most ancient and sacred text of Hinduism. The study of *Ayurveda* is traditionally divided into eight sections: (1) general principles, (2) pathology, (3) the basis of diagnosis, (4) physiology, (5) prognosis, (6) therapeutics, (7) pharmaceutics, and (8) texts on successful treatment. The curriculum thus far seems very like that of Western medicine;

however, closely integrated with these subjects are practices of religious devotion and yoga that uniquely differentiate them.

The Three Primary Humors

Health is considered to be maintained by the balance of three primary humors: wind (*vāyu*), gall (*pitta*), and mucus (*kapha*). The basic theory is that the combination of the elements earth and water give rise to *kapha,* the mixing of fire and earth gives rise to *pitta,* and the combining of ether and air results in *vāyu*. In this model there are in all five separate winds or "breaths" by which the various body functions are controlled. Consciousness is said to reside in the heart (as the mind was said to reside in the heart in the Chinese paradigm), not in the brain.

The Bases of Diagnoses

Through the practice of hatha yoga a considerable amount of knowledge was amassed about the neurology of the body. Throughout Ayurvedic literature there is a firm realization that the functions of the body are based on natural law, particularly laws concerned with cycles. Man is looked upon as a microcosm of the universe in whose being is reflected the functionings of the macrocosm, the universe. It is recognized that the individual is the cause of his or her own illness through karmic law and, therefore, must accept personal responsibility for the maintenance of health. Strong emphasis is placed on diet for health maintenance. Climatic changes are looked upon seriously as both the cause and cure of certain illnesses. A prime consideration in this concern is the determination of the type of climatic conditions in which the individual grew up and any change in these conditions that are concomitants of the illness. An individual's mental attitude, particularly toward morals, is stressed as the underlying condition for psychosomatic illnesses.

The fundamental principles of *Ayurveda* concern the five basic elements of the universe (which, as noted above, are ruled by the Dhyāni Buddhas), the three humors (the *tridoshas*), and the seven constituents of the body. The perspective of body functioning is that when food is assimilated it becomes successively food juice, blood, flesh, fat, bone, marrow, and semen. It is said that semen (females are also said to have semen) is a "vital juice" that tones the whole body.

When a humor (*dosa*) is out of balance, it essentially means that it is no longer in the appropriate proportion to the other humors. The harmonic interaction among the humors underlies proper body functioning. The goal of administering drugs or herbal preparations is to lessen that imbalance. The humor that is in disequilibrium will affect one or more of the seven body components. Interpretations of both illnesses and cures are closely associated with religion and ritual.

The Relationship of the Three Body Types to the Three Humors

Basic to the diagnosis is the theory that there are three body types which correlate in a one-to-one fashion with the three humors. The *dosa* or humor that predominates at an individual's time of conception specifies the body type for that individual's lifetime. In general, the body type defines the individual's physical and psychological traits, with definite patterns in diet, personal habits, and the like being attributed to each body type. Intervening factors are race, ethnic origin, the seasons, hereditary factors, the environment, and other special considerations.

The Examination of the Pulse

An examination of the pulse, somewhat similar to that of the Chinese, has been added in the last three centuries. The quality of the pulse is related to the three humors in this fashion:

> Usually the *vayu* (wind) type pulse is described as having a snake-like motion; the *pitta* (gall) type pulse has a jumping action similar to that of a frog; the *kapha* (mucus) type pulse moves slowly and steadily like an elephant or swan.[19]

Individual and the Disease Evaluated as a Whole

Each of the body types has a different reaction to drugs and treatment, so that not only must the medication be individually prescribed, but each patient must be examined, and also the patient and the disease process itself must be evaluated as a whole. The examination is done in three ways, always in reference to the principle of macrocosm-microcosm ("as above, so below"): (1) by practical (*i.e.,* observable) methods; (2) in accordance with the teachings of learned sages; and (3) by analogy. Ayurvedic thought emphasized the importance of a highly developed sense of intuition in the practitioner.

Summary

In summary, we see a system of thought somewhat reminiscent of the Chinese, but perhaps the confrontation with the universal forces is more personal within the Indian paradigm. The conception of psychic states and states of consciousness after death is more richly organized. Most importantly, there is a deep embedment of and reference to both the disease and its cure. Underlying it all is a unitive sense of relationship of all people:

To but one goal are marching everywhere
All human beings, though they may seem to walk
Divergent paths; and that Goal is I.
                                        Bhagavad Gita

References

1. Bashan WL: The practice of medicine in ancient and medieval India. In Leslie C (ed): Asian Medical Systems, pp 18–19. Berkeley, University of California Press, 1976
2. Chatterji JC: The Wisdom of the Vedas, p 28. Wheaton, Theosophical Publishing House, Quest Book Reprint, 1973
3. Chatterji, *op cit*, pp 27–38
4. Woodroffe J: The Serpent Fire, p 105. Madras, Ganesh, 1964
5. Riviere JM: Tantrik Yoga, p 38 London, Rider, *n.d.*
6. Eliade M: Yoga: Immortality and Freedom, p 246. Princeton, Princeton University Press (Bollingen Series LVI), 1969; see also Evans-Wentz WY: Tibetan Yoga and Secret Doctrines, pp 192–195. London, Oxford University Press, 1967
7. Evans-Wentz WY: Tibet's Great Yogi Milrepa, p ix. London, Oxford University Press, 1959
8. Govinda A: Creative Meditation and Multidimensional Consciousness, p 71. Wheaton, Theosophical Publishing House, 1976
9. Eliade, *op cit*, pp 241–245
10. Yü LK: The Secrets of Chinese Meditation. London, Rider, 1964
11. Krishna G: Kundalini: the Evolutionary Energy in Man. Berkeley, Shambala, 1970
12. Evans-Wentz, Tibetan Yoga, *op cit*, pp 335–338
13. Eliade, Yoga, *op cit*, pp 12–13
14. Eliade, Yoga, *loc cit*
15. Evans-Wentz WY (trans): Tibetan Book of the Dead, 3rd ed. London, Oxford University Press, 1957
16. Harding ME: Psychic Energy: Its Source and Its Transformation, p 277. Princeton, Princeton University Press (Bollingen Series X), 1973
17. Jung CG: Psychological commentary. In Evans-Wentz WY: (trans): The Tibetan Book of the Dead, 3rd ed, p xiv. London, Oxford University Press, 1957
18. Durant W, Durant A: The Story of Civilization. I. Our Indian Heritage. New York, Simon & Schuster, 1952
19. Thakkur CG: Introduction to Ayurveda, p 129. New York, Asi Publications, 1974

5 The Mediterranean Sphere of Influence

The Mediterranean Sea acted as a basin toward which flowed many cultures. The exotic life-styles and profound philosophies of the diverse ethnic groups that lined its shores provided vital currents of new ideas that overflowed and in time nourished the growth and development of European thought. A major contributor was the rich delta empire of Egypt, whose dynasties arose out of the mythic past of earliest times, but whose reality persisted until the third century A.D.

The Egyptian Influence

Egypt was a land of ritual and magic with a strange preoccupation with death. The craft of mummification, however, gave those who plied that trade an advanced understanding of the human body. The knowledge of the Egyptians reached beyond the simple delta confines, nurturing first the provinces and then the centers of Greek thought. There, through the genius of Galen, knowledge about the human body was reorganized and integrated into European thought for hundreds of years.

Egyptian Holism Described in Myth

An intrinsic holism wells up from Egyptian thought at about the time of the Third Dynasty. It is described in myth that in the beginning there was no form or structure; all was chaos. Chaos was depicted as an ocean or shapeless magma called *Nun*, which contained the potential for life. Within this inchoate state was a conscious principle that has existence even in the most ancient past. This principle, or god, was *Atum*. Atum is the conscious principle and his name means "the whole" or "the complete."

Atum was able to fertilize himself and to thus produce Shu and Tefnut, who became the first divine couple. Shu represented the air,

which was recognized as the prime life-giving substance. His consort,
Tefnut, represented the water or moisture in the atmosphere. From their
union came Geb, who became earth-god, and Nut, the sky-goddess.
From Geb and Nut were born Osiris and Isis, and Seth and Nephthys.
The latter were gods of the earth itself and therefore were earthbound.[1]

The Nile—Source of the Mystical Nature of Periodic Renewal

Through the ebb and flow of the Nile, around which Egyptian life
centered, came a knowledge of the mystical nature of cyclic
phenomena, such as periodic renewal. This concept of rebirth became a
central tenet of the Egyptians' belief systems and was extended to the
death and reincarnation of human beings.

The Practice of Necropsy

A constructive understanding of the healing and health of the body
came out of the practice of necropsy, the study of the dead, and the
practice of mummification. This aspect was particularly well developed
as early as 3000 b.c. under Imhotep, the chief physician to Zoser,
Pharoah of the Third Dynasty. Imhotep was deified after his own death
and his tomb became a pilgrimage site.

The Hathors, Egyptian Nurses of the Newborn

Nursing in ancient Egypt was activated under the guise of a sometimes
terrifying but usually helpful goddess named Hathor. In particular, this
goddess was the protector of infants and was present with her helpers
at the birth of the pharaohs. Egyptian nurses of the newborn were
known as the Hathors. Their particular charge was the development of
the *Ka*, the nonobservable replica of the physical body. The *Ka* was the
source of all attributes and delimitations of the physical body, such as
illness.

Illnesses of the Mummies

Studies of the remains of entombed mummies have revealed several
illnesses that besieged the ancient Egyptians. Schistosome eggs (which
produce flukes, a trematode worm that is parasitic in man) and
atheromatous changes in the arteries of a 3000-year-old mummy were
noted in an early study.[2] Evidence of tuberculosis, tapeworms, filarial
elephantiasis, and ectoparasites were found in a later study.[3] Other
studies on mummies have found that rickets, iron-deficiency anemia
associated with parasitism, and pellagra were common among ancient
Egyptians. There also is considerable documentation of childhood

protein-deficiency syndromes that apparently were the sequelae of severe gastrointestinal and respiratory infections. Eye infections, particularly trachoma, were also common.

The After-Death State as a Continuum of Consciousness

Ancient Egyptian thought, like those of the Chinese and the Indian, considered life and the after-death state to be a continuum of consciousness. Daily activities of the ancient Egyptians were influenced importantly by the felt presence of the divine in their pharaohs and in the natural elements. They were deeply embued with a need for ritual and magic, perhaps to control themselves on the one hand and to control nature on the other. These needs produced a distinctive psychological unity among the people of the Old Kingdom. Egyptian literature on ritual and magic dates back to the Fifth Dynasty, about 2000 B.C.

The Egyptian Book of the Dead

Much energy went into the study of death and the afterlife. The major papyrus, called today *The Egyptian Book of the Dead* or *The Coming Forth From the Day*, is a detailed account of life after death. In it are specific instructions for the use of *Ka*.[4] One might therefore say that it was the earliest text on nursing!

Egypt, as the hub of the Mediterranean world, influenced people from the many nations that came to her ports. Greece was so influenced as a civilization, particularly from the time of Alexander the Great in the third century B.C. Alexander spent many years studying the contents of the great Egyptian libraries in what came to be known as Alexandria. In time, however, Egypt's powerful influence waned, and the Mediterranean center of culture shifted to Greece.

The Greek Influence

Traces of Shamanistic Ideology in Myths of Ancient Greece

In early Grecian myth one can see traces of shamanistic ideology. There is, for instance, direct reference to the notion of "soul travel" (see Chap. 2) in the myth of Orpheus in which Orpheus descends into Hades to recover the soul of his wife, Eurydice. According to this myth, Orpheus had both healing ability and the power of divination. He played a lyre and his songs had a magical power. The whole of nature was affected by his music. Wild animals were said to follow him, the trees leaned toward him, and the souls of fierce men were said to become gentle when they heard his music.

Plato expressed a belief in an after-life. In his *Republic,* he writes that Er, the son of Armenios, was killed on the battelfield, but he returned to life on the twelfth day, after his body had already been placed on the funeral pyre. Then Er recounted to others the visions of the afterlife world that he said he was shown. It is thought that Er was in a cataleptic-like trance which outwardly resembles that of the shaman.[5]

Pythagoras, the learned sage who attracted many of the most brilliant minds of his era (fifth century B.C.), was also said to have descended into Hades. He, too, had a clear sense of the continuum of life. In words attributed to him, he taught as follows:[6]

> Old age is not to be considered with reference
> to an egress from the present life, but the
> beginning of a blessed one.
> Death and decay are part of the natural process
> of change and mutability,
> Which pertains only to things which are
> unreal,
> And by which all things are renewed and restored
> to balance

Cyclic Phenomena as Natural Law

The sense of cyclic phenomena as natural law comes through very clearly in Greek thought. The Greeks, in fact, had a word, *chronos,* to indicate recurring events. Chronos was the Greek god of time, and he was said to have been born of Gaia, Mother Earth, and Uranus, Father of the Heavens. In this way, father related to son that time derives from the relative positions of earth and other heavenly bodies. It was to wrest this secret from nature that astrology and astronomy played such an important part in ancient cultures.

Historically, the appropriate use of time for healthful living and the rationale for Greek therapeutics were firmly based on the study of natural cycles. Specific timed routines were devised for the intake of nutrients and herbal medications. Various therapeutic procedures, such as baths, massage, and so on, were set for different times of day, night, and seasons. Hippocrates counseled physicians to note carefully any signs of irregularity in the habits of their patients, for irregularity denoted ill health.

Incubation, the Study of Healing Dreams

The study of healing dreams and visions through autosuggestion and hypnosis was well known in China, India, and the Mediterranean countries. This form of therapeutics was a forerunner of modern analytic psychology and autogenic and biofeedback training.

For the early Greeks, dreams were regarded as memories of events that had actually happened and, therefore, much time was given to creating circumstances which would encourage dreaming. Certain rites, called *incubation* (from *incubare,* to sleep in a sacred place), induced a deep hypnagogic state during which the unconscious could be directed toward the healing of one's bodily ills. Meier, in his classic modern interpretation of incubation, concluded that the efficacy of this therapeutic method confirmed a basic tenet of the ancient world that "... bodily sickness and psychic defects were ... an inseparable unity." He also makes clear that symptoms were the *coniunctio naturae,* the experienced point of correspondence between the inner world and the outer, in what would be described today in Jungian terms as an act of synchronicity.[7]

The Asclepian Sanctuaries

In ancient Greece the rites of incubation took place in the Asclepian sanctuaries. More than 400 of these were built during the 1000-year span of the worship of Asclepius as the heroic protector and healer, from about 500 B.C. to 500 A.D. The myths say that Asclepius learned the mysteries of healing from Chiron, the centaur. Asclepius was very successful in his cures and finally even brought people who had seemingly died back to life. For so interfering with the divine order of things, Zeus killed him with a thunderbolt fashioned by Cyclops. After his death, Asclepius became a hero and was able to work miracles.

One of the forms that Asclepius took was that of a serpent or snake, and statues show him holding a staff on which a snake is entwined. This staff and snake representation became the basis for the *caduceus,* the emblem of the physician today. For the ancient Greeks it symbolized *kundalini* (see Chap. 4), a symbol of consciousness and the renewal of life.

The ritual of the Asclepian sanctuaries required that the ill person first be called to healing in some decisive manner, either through an irresistible impulse that could not be denied or through a dream. Upon arrival he or she underwent a cleansing bath and then made a sacrifice to the god Asclepius. The sick person then was led to the *aboton,* the innermost sanctuary, to sleep on a *cline,* a couch (from which came the word "clinic"). Significantly, the patient had to have the *right* dream in order for this therapy to be effective, and the right dream brought an instantaneous cure. Meier writes that frequently the god Asclepius touched the affected part of the patient in the dream. Everyone who was thus cured through dreams had to record the dreams—thus building a body of clinical texts—and then gave an offering in appreciation.[8]

The Organization of Health Practices by Galen

Mediterranean thought on health practices was so decisively and comprehensively organized by Galen that its influence extended from about the second century A.D. through the Middle Ages in both Christian and Islamic countries. Galen's writings clearly state his relationship to the therapeutics of the ancient Greeks, calling himself the "therapeut" of his "fatherly god, Asclepius." A major approach used by Galen in his teachings was that appropriate treament for the ill should be based on analogical thinking.

Humoral Pathology as the Basis of the Galenic System

The primary tenets of the Galenic system were based upon humoral pathology, which had originated in the Hippocratic school of Kos and was modified by Aristotle. The four major humors were blood, mucus, yellow bile, and black bile. The four primary qualities were warmth (heat), cold, moisture (or dampness), and dryness. In essence, this statement of humors strongly resembles that of both Chinese and Indian thought. Galen's interpretation of these qualities was that mucus was damp and cold, blood was damp and hot, yellow bile was dry and hot, and black bile was damp and cold. Also to be taken into consideration were certain external factors, such as the climate, the patient's age, profession, and habits, and the customs of his or her culture. All of this, too, is reminiscent of both Chinese and Indian thought.

The dominance of one of the four humors importantly influenced the person's complexion, personal habits, and also "temperament," which could be sanguine, phlegmatic, choleric, or melancholic. A law of opposites was inherent in the Galenic system of treatments, so that "hot" diseases were treated by "cold" remedies, moist by dry, and so forth, in a logic based on symmetry.

Galen's Treatment of Psychosomatic Illness

Galen had profound insight into psychosomatic problems. A story is told about how he cured a patient who had the delusion that he had swallowed a snake. Galen had the patient fully describe the incident and the snake, and then he obtained such a snake. His treatment was most direct: first, he blindfolded the patient and then gave him a powerful emetic. When the blindfolded patient vomited, Galen placed the snake in the vomited material and then removed the patient's blindfold. The patient saw the snake in that condition, was satisfied that it was the snake he envisioned he had swallowed, and his symptoms and fears disappeared.

Pythagorean Theories on Music Therapy

Galenic ideas continued to be influential until medieval times. Ideas of other Greeks, such as Pythagoras' theories relative to both mathematics and to the use of music to create or change emotional mood, also influenced medieval thought through the works of Isidore of Seville (fourth century A.D.), Cassiodorus (fifth century, A.D.), and Boethius (fifth century A.D.). The famous *Treatise on Music* by Boethius, who based his theory on the works of Pythagoras, was routinely used at Italian medical universities. One of the famous musical therapies was for sciatica and back pain. In the sixteenth century, the plastic surgeon Tagliacozzi stimulated a resurgence of interest in the concept of music therapy by using it both preoperatively and postoperatively for his patients. Much to his credit, he also advocated the therapeutic use of diet.[9]

The Study of Pulses Under Galen

The study of pulses entered Europe through Galen's 16 books on pulse, in which he distinguished 27 distinct types of pulse—a 15-fold bit of one-upmanship over the Chinese, so to speak!

Elaborate mathematical theories on pulse beat evolved that were based on music theory and a learned sense of touch in relation to rhythm, proportion, and meter. In fact, pulse was thought to demonstrate the fundamental nature of music, since both pulse and music are characterized by rhythmic patterns of time intervals. This recognition of a significant correlation between music and physiologic acts comes very close to current research findings.

Today it is understood that our every rhythmic act of daily living has specific limits of frequency per second, the upper range or highest frequency being approximately 7 cycles per second, with a minimum individual deviation of 2 cycles per second. These figures hold for such common activities as chewing, tapping, and walking, and for all routine and repetitive functions. It is of interest that this "biological resonance" is hypothesized to be of fundamental importance in the response of human beings to music that has a pronounced beat, such as jazz or rock music. Sollberger, who has done extensive research on biorhythms, states the following:

> One may, of course, speculate why so-called "primitive" music achieves such an immediate response in the unprejudiced listener through its rhythm and why the frequency lies in the region of

muscle reflex action. Some kind of biological resonance would be a good guess.[10]

The Renaissance

The Renaissance Concept of the Universal Man

With the full blossoming of the Renaissance the concept of the universal man arose. The universal man was one within whom many talents and interests were finely integrated in a holistic manner. This was the emergence of the concept of *uomo unico* in fourteenth century Italy. This unique person, the man or woman of extensive interests and vast knowledge, was looked upon as the epitome of human development. Typified by such figures as Michelangelo, da Vinci and Dante, these persons had remarkable range to their abilities as poet, philosopher, artist, scientist, engineer, inventor, artisan, and seer, and each seemed to encompass a vision of infinite human potential.[11]

The Holism of the Early Christian Mystics

In quite another fashion, Christian mystics such as St. Francis of Assisi and Meister Eckhart contributed considerably to the concept of holism by speaking clearly and publicly to the actuality of the individual and God meeting in direct and intimate experience. For Eckhart this personal and courageous declaration meant excommunication from the Roman Catholic Church.[12] However, one must also note that the churches and other holy places of the Middle Ages also offered sanctuaries, sacred retreats, and the catharsis of the confessional as healing measures.

The Decline of Holism and the Rise of Cartesian Dualism

By the sixteenth century the concept of holism in the Western world gets cloudy with other concerns. The dualistic view of "mind" and "matter" as separate entities gained prominence and popularity, influenced by philosopher René Descartes. With the forced bifurcation of mind and matter, a rational but reductionistic and mechanistic view of man and the universe emerged. This simplistic perspective, in vogue until quite recently, compartmentalized facts about the details of the universe, and then categorized "the details of the details," as Thomas puts it.[13] This delimitation has a persistent tendency to make us very knowledgeable about a few carefully demarcated things in our universe while we remain ignorant about the context as a living, vital whole.

Summary

We have seen that the evolution of Western thought on health practices within a holistic framework arose from the Mediterranean basin to decisively influence the thinking of the Greeks and, through their genius, the rest of the Western world.

Several similarities exist among Chinese, Indian, and Mediterranean holistic thought, as illustrated in Figure 5-1. They all share the concept of microcosm–macrocosm, which establishes the basic holism, the existence of nonobservable dimensions of the physical body which intimately influence physical and psychological health and indicate a fuller human scope than we currently acknowledge. Within this perspective must be included the concept of life as a continuum in

Fig. 5–1.
A symbolic representation by D. Krieger of the integration of the ancient and contemporary. In this mandala is a central axis of signs. Uppermost on this axis is the Indian symbol for Ākasha, the Continuum. In the middle is the symbol for the principle of macrocosm–microcosm: as above, so below. The lower symbol on the central axis depicts the Chinese concept of the *yin–yang* complementarity. The signs on the lateral axes represent (from *left to right* and from *top to bottom*) the elements of fire, air, earth, and water as they are currently written in the modern languages of physics and chemistry.

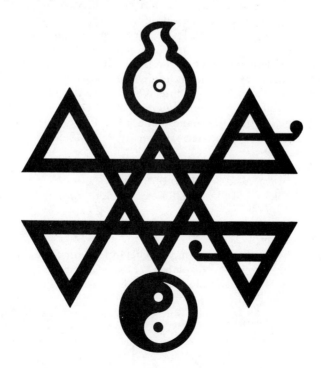

which death is an extended state of consciousness that can be experienced in a knowledgeable fashion (even as late as the Middle Ages the craft of dying was carefully described in the medieval opus *De Arte Moriende*).

There is also the persistent theory of specific humors or elements whose balanced proportions are central to the maintenance of health, the prevention of disease, the restoration of physiologic and psychological harmony, and finally, and importantly, the crucial nature of the maintenance of a well-balanced, unitive relationship with the environment.

The similar world view of these three great cultures, which shared time frames but were significantly removed from one another spatially, lends credence to the notion that this holistic world view was so completely a shared knowledge because it was the outgrowth of natural law in the lives of people who lived in direct touch with nature. This natural experience uninterrupted by intellectual rationalizations was the common tie among them. Because they lived the experience, they knew.

References

1. Grimal P (ed): Larousse World Mythology, pp 30–31. London, Paul Hamlyn, 1972
2. Ruffer MA: Notes on the presence of Bilharzia Haemotobia in Egyptian mummies of the 12th Dynasty, 1250–1000 B.C. Br Med J 1:16, 1914
3. Sandison AT: Parasitic diseases. In Brothwell AT, Sandison D: Diseases in Antiquity: a Survey of the Diseases, Injuries and Surgery of Early Populations, pp 178–188. Springfield, Charles C Thomas, 1967
4. Tirard HM: The Egyptian Book of the Dead, pp 48–49. London, Rider, 1910
5. Eliade M: Shamanism: Archaic Techniques of Ecstasy, p 393. Princeton, Princeton University Press (Bollingen Series LXXVI), 1964
6. Huson H: Pythagoron, p 31. *Privately published*, 1947
7. Meier CA: Ancient Incubation and Modern Psychotherapy. Translated by M Curtis. Evanston, Northwestern University Press, 1968
8. Meier, *op cit*, p 59
9. Cosman MP, Chandler B (eds): Marchant's world: science in the fourteenth century. Ann NY Acad Sci 314:6, 1978
10. Sollberger A: Biological Rhythms Research, p 136. Amsterdam, Elsevier, 1965
11. Burckhardt J: The Civilization of the Renaissance in Italy, pp 129 *et seq*. New York, Macmillan, 1921
12. Skorpen E: The whole man. Main Currents in Modern Thought 32, Nos. 2–5:79 (Retrospective issue, November 17, 1940–November 17, 1975)
13. Thomas L: The Medusa and the Snail, p 7. New York, Viking, 1979

Part 2
An Overview of Modern Holistic Health Practices

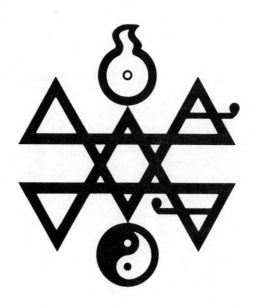

6 The Contemporary Holistic Health Perspective

In order to gain a perspective on contemporary holistic health practices, it may be useful to resort to a principle that is central in cultures that have based their world view on holism. This is the principle of macrocosm–microcosm. For this purpose let us focus attention on the works of Beals, who studied the strategies of people who, faced by illness, are looking for cures.[1] Beals' study was on a small but populous corner of the world, South India. Reflected in this concentrated microcosm are issues that underlie the search for health common to all people in our time. Beals found a large array of health practitioners who were chosen according to several factors.

The primary factor in choosing a health practitioner was the concept of the problem as the person perceived it within the pattern of strategies used in other aspects of the person's life-style. This pattern was most frequently concerned with the maintenance of individual harmony with the laws of the universe as that person understood them to be. Therefore, prayer, worship, and magic were resorted to, as well as modern scientific methods.

Of secondary importance in choosing a health practitioner was the kind of disease that was present. This was important because the type of illness gave cues as to whether the illness came from natural or supernatural sources.

The folk interpretation of the sickness was a third criterion. If the illness was caused by sin, one could expect punishment. If the illness was the result of an attack by spirits, psychological illness or death would ensue. If, however, the illness was due to "bad" or impure blood, a dietary imbalance was implied and there was the possibility of easy cure.

The next priority in choosing a health practitioner was the economic and social status of the family. The loss of working time was of concern here. An additional concern was the amount of money charged by the practitioner. Therefore, the first choice was for treatment by those who knew spells or home treatment. Western medicine was expensive; on the other hand, it also was more prestigious.

Finally, the kinds of advice and information available at the time a strategy was adopted were crucial. The first impulse would be to "keep quiet" in the hope that the illness would disappear. A secondary strategy was to ask the advice of relatives, friends, and neighbors. If there was agreement on the diagnosis and the treatment, the ill person was given home remedies. It was known, however, that certain illnesses were treated best by certain doctors. Western medical doctors were known to treat best those whose illnesses required antibiotics, chemotherapy, or surgery. In the case of natural causes of illness such as snakebite, reliance was placed on the expertise of traditional curers.

If there was some shame attached to the problem, such as with impotence, prestigious licensed practitioners were not consulted. In all cases where there was no fixed strategy, the easiest and least expensive treatments were used first. In times of epidemics, Beals says that the villagers accepted all treatments that were offered.

Within this framework, any of the following health practitioners might be chosen, and frequently the ill person consulted more than one simultaneously. The choices included local healers; saints and religious figures; priests, ministers, and missionaries; drug and herb specialists; midwives and persons "that had the gift"; astrologers and diviners; and ayurvedic doctors and Western medical doctors.

Although this study took place in small villages, it can readily be seen that the villagers' responses to illness are basically similar to those of the most intelligent city sophisticates in that they are very human reactions in the face of crisis.

The Beginning of the Modern Holistic Approach

Particularly in the second half of the twentieth century there has been an unprecedented intermix among people of dissimilar cultures that has served to level out differences. This has been fostered and even accelerated by rapid advances in the technology of communications and travel, as well as by a significant general increase in worldwide standards of living. Also, there are illnesses that all people share, many of which result from and at the same time alter their life-style. By far the most common of these is the epidemic of stress-related illnesses that know no geographic boundaries. There is little relief from the frenetic pace of modern living and its cumulative stresses, whether one lives in the midst of the current post-technological effort or on its fringes. The physiologic reactions to these stresses have run the gamut from migraine headache to cardiac dysfunction, depending on how the clustering of physiologic reactivities pattern themselves in the individual.

The revolutions of the 1960s were to a great extent psychosocial in nature and represented a desperate attempt to break out of this life-wasting mold into a more life-affirmative and individually assertive stance. It was a time of mass confrontation and reexamination of life-styles and world view. The repercussions were felt in the farthermost reaches of the world, wherever the thrust of modern communications and travel made its impact.

There were many responses to this impact. Where the response was positive, people who had previously felt nothing but a sense of overwhelming powerlessness in the face of impossible personal, social, and economic situations began to use the wealth of technological advances such as facilitated communication and travel to critically change their psychological perspective and social conditions. Out of this mélange arose concepts of living that were viable alternatives to the previously accepted modes of living. From the pool of ideas concerning the well-being of the individual developed a loosely defined notion of practices. Because they added to the individual's knowledge of how to use himself or herself as an actualized being, the practices adhered to the concept of holism and became known as holistic health practices.

A significant difference in perspective between the methods of Western medicine and a transcultural approach to health became readily apparent. This differentiation has been cogently stated by Sobel:

> Western scientific medicine is largely concerned with objective, nonpersonal, physicochemical explanations of disease as well as its technical control . . . (whereas) . . . Traditional healing techniques are armed principally at providing meaningful and understandable explanations of the illness experience.[2]

Historically, one of the potent forces that turned people in the United States away from the accepted dependence on Western medicine was the decision which originated in, and was endorsed by, the American Medical Association. This decision raised considerably the costs of medical care just before a federally supported program to alleviate the heavy burden of medical costs on the elderly went into effect. Concomitantly, several previously unknown or ignored facts about significant negative effects of Western medicine made their way into the popular press and served to accelerate the search for alternative methods of health care. For instance, one of the bits of information concerned the frightening effects of pharmacologic dependence for extended periods of time. The indirect and delayed side-effects that accompanied prolonged dependence on drugs and frequently led to iatrogenic disease (that is, disease caused by the medical treatment itself) led many people to explore alternative methods of health care.

There also has been an increase in the general level of

sophistication of people as a result of a trend toward the continuance of higher education, and with it a more discriminating sense of choice in the care of their bodies. Access to diverse literature has given the general public a more eclectic appreciation for the findings of other cultures and a deeper understanding of the growing edge of Western cultural mores. One insight that has caused persons in the holistic health movement to look again at the age-old theory of the humors has been the realization that the doctrine of the balance of the humors has been restated in our time in reference to chemical and hormonal processes. Penetrating discernments such as this have coupled with other knowledge that our post-technological body of information has made clear for us. An example of the latter is that at the level of elementary particles, matter and energy become indistinguishable (a recognition which has confronted the best minds since Einstein first stated it at the beginning of the twentieth century, but which few could interpret to lay people until recently). These discernments and post-technological information have armed the imagnination of the multitudes with the possibility of a rationale for the wisdom of the ancients. On the negative side, this has given rise to a mere use of terms within the holistic health movement without an understanding of their semantics. On the positive side, however, immense strides have been taken in research which has attempted to synthesize transcultural knowledges about human well-being with contemporary information about the human condition. In thus combining even the extreme edges of the spectrum of human thought through the ages, more often than not it has been found that there is more that is similar rather than dissimilar among the minds of men of all literate times regarding man's interaction with the universe.

This common, human linkage of ideas arrested the attention of Jung, whose writings speak fluently to the psychological analysis of our time. In writing a commentary on an ancient Eastern text, Jung specifically notes the commonality of all thought.[3] He speaks of the more than five decades in which he conducted his life work, during which he had no more than a most superficial idea of Chinese philosophy. He had discovered in the later years of his life that the psychological techniques he had developed for his patients were remarkably similar to those that had been developed by the best minds of the East. He developed a striking analogy that could also be an assumption for the above-noted modern synthesis of the ancient and the contemporary knowledges about the well-being of humans that underlie holistic health practices. Jung says:

> . . . just as the human body shows a common anatomy over and above racial differences, so too does the psyche possess a common substratum.[4]

It is within this context that contemporary holistic health practices should be evaluated.

A Generalized Modeling of Suffering and Illness

Holistic health practices are based on alternative rather than traditional ways of perceiving illness. Within this general modeling it is useful to consider Durckheim's overview of human suffering and illness, which he perceives as being of two types:

> . . . that engendered by functional impairment and having mundane implications; and that caused by "not being at one with the Self", i.e., not to be what one actually is.[5]

The former is concerned with some disabling effect that prohibits the person from meeting his or her responsibilities to society and from taking advantage of the opportunities offered by society. "Something is lacking," he says, "with respect to that which one has, knows or is able to do." The differentiating quality of the latter category is that it is concerned with a personal deficit, a lack with respect ot the inner being of the self, ". . . to what one *is*."

At its base, the difference depends on whether the ill person is concerned with being unable to function in outer society or is concerned about a personal inability to attain self-realization. Durckheim's point is that the former, more pragmatic objective has been the goal of traditional therapies, whereas the latter has sought the goal of a wholeness of being. The holistic mode in actuality enhances the integration of both of these extremes, he conlcudes, for ". . . in the end only a person who has come to an understanding with himself can enter into an understanding with the world."[6]

The General Orientation to Holistic Health Practices

The underlying premise of holistic health practices is that it is a major misconception of our times that the germ theory accounts for all illness. In actuality, it is established fact—depending upon which source you read—that between 50% and 80% of all illness is psychosomatic in origin.[7] This means that illness is the product of a complementary interaction between mind and body under conditions of stress that cannot be reconciled. The goal of the holistic perspective is to treat all aspects of the person's problems by an integrated approach that considers both the person in the context of the problem and the problem in the context of the uniqueness of the individual, thus giving the situation a more humanistic orientation than has previously been the case.

A very important point arises from this last consideration. It now becomes clear that the perspective to treating illness should not be that the illness falls into the domain of one therapist alone. Rather, the patient's acceptance of responsibility for the illness or wellness of his or her being is crucial to healing, to prevention of illness, and to the maintenance of high-level well-being. Within this context the therapist and the client are seen to be partners; the client actively participates in the therapeutic stance as an actualizer of health potential. Illness need no longer carry a negative connotation. It can be seen as a limitation and an opportunity to learn more about the fullness of self. This last has been the underlying stimulus to the explosion of growth experiences and encounters with personal values that have been pursued by the consumer of holistic health practices during the past decade. Finally, in order to be an intelligent and understanding participant in this therapeutic process, the therapist must have insight into his or her own self from this multivariate point of view.

The Major Avenues of Holistic Health Practices

Hypnosis

As was noted earlier, hypnotic suggestion, as in temple sleep, was used therapeutically in ancient times in India, Egypt, and Greece (see Chap. 5). Its more recent use for migraine headache, severe burns, asthma, and sexual dysfunction has been of varying interest to therapists over the past two hundred years.[8]

Recently, Hilgard of Stanford University, in studies on hypnotic analgesia, found that there seems to be more than one dimension of awareness that operates even when a person has been deeply hypnotized. He has called this coextensive consciousness "the hidden observer."[9] In his studies, Hilgard has found that the hidden observer escaped his attempts to place it in a passive hypnotic state and, instead, did such left hemisphere tasks as the working out of statistical problems and the analysis of observations. One of the useful aspects of this finding has been introduced into the use of hypnosis for the relief of pain in patients with terminal cancer. The purpose in this therapy is to call attention to the hidden observer that can be otherwise occupied even in the face of pain. Thus the patients can experience for themselves that they are more complex and complete than that aspect that is involved with the pain. In this way, patients are encouraged to actualize more of their potential in the service of the therapeutic process.

Autogenic Training

Autogenic training, a direct relation of clinical hypnosis, was developed by Johannes Schultz, a psychiatrist, in the 1930s in Germany. Its major ploy is to dampen response to external stimuli and to heighten an inward focusing of attention. This serves to alter the state of consciousness so that a deep relaxation accompanies a somewhat dissociative frame of mind.

Autogenic training is done in either a reclining or a relaxed sitting position, with the mind in a passive, almost casual and nonexpectant attitutde. A series of commands to the person's physical body then follows, the commands being stereotyped and impersonal, although said by the subject. The series starts with the dominant hand. While paying passive attention to the hand, one repeats to one's self the statement "My (dominant) hand is heavy." This is repeated at the rate of about six times per minute. Then passive attention is given the other hand and the procedure is repeated. When the feeling of heaviness has been adequately experienced in both hands, attention is given to doing the procedure with both arms at the same time. Attention is next gently focused on the legs: first one, then the other, then both, until a generalized sense of heaviness is felt throughout the body. This process of autosuggestion is then continued. Instead of heaviness, however, the person focuses on feelings of warmth in the extremities. Using the pattern noted above, the person says "My (dominant) hand is warm," and continues the progression in the extremities. It is important to tell the body to stop these procedures, and so a convention is adopted to clearly state "Arms firm, breathe deeply, open eyes" in an affirmative voice after each repetition.

Luthe, a student of Schultz, developed a number of exercises that have become standard. He gives instructions for heart regulation ("Heartbeat calm and regular," terminated with "Eyes open, breathe deeply"), respiratory exercises ("It breathes me," followed by "Eyes open, breathe deeply"), and for acquiring a sensation of warmth in the abdomen ("My solar plexus is warm," followed by "Eyes open, breathe deeply"). Finally one tells one's self "My forehead is cool" in the same manner, thus completing the physical exercises. These exercises, incidentally, are given over a period of several weeks' training, usually with a certified trainer in attendance.

The deep relaxation and regulation when acquired are said to be transferable to other physiologic states that are amenable to autosuggestion so that they can return to a normal range of harmonic self-regulation.[10]

Biofeedback

Biofeedback has been called the yoga of the West. It stems from the work of Miller of Rockefeller University, who, through systematic rewards and punishments, was able to demonstrate that mice can be conditioned to control functions of the autonomic nervous system that previously had been thought to be beyond voluntary control.[11] Biofeedback has taught human beings to also develop this type of voluntary control. By learning to pick up subtle cues from their bodies, people can learn to control normally unconscious functions.

The methods of choice are to actuate a visible or audible signal to inform the subject whether or not he or she is in fact controlling a certain function on command. This feedback serves to teach the person the right responses, and to repeat the controlled action until it can be done at will. It seems that any aspect of the autonomic nervous system can be controlled under these circumstances, particularly cardiovascular problems, chronic pain such as migraine headache, and problems due to stress-related illnesses.

The secret of biofeedback is to greatly magnify the physiologic response and display it to the subject so he or she can know that, when an effort was made, it proceeded in the correct direction. Biofeedback can control response either within the body structure or outside of the body on the skin. Green and Green of the Menninger Institute have done extensive research on biofeedback. Their theory is that control of energies both within and outside of the body can occur ". . . only after we become conscious of our unconscious."[12]

Reports on the use of electromyography biofeedback for muscle reeducation in persons who have had cardiovascular accidents, Bell's palsy, or cerebral palsy have been very heartening and decisive in considerably altering rehabilitation goals.[13] There also has been a strong interest in biofeedback among educators. Significant improvement in focus of attention, emotional stability, and communications and reading skills have been reported, as has a reduction in anxiety and hyperactive behavior in students.[14]

Guided Imagery

The study of imagery, although probably one of humanity's earliest tools of communication to self and to others, has been very little studied in this century. In its current definition, imagery encompasses more than mere visualization. Imagery includes internal behavior, such as internalized sounds, feelings, words, symbols, and subtle body sensations.

Guided imagery, in which either a therapist, a tape-recorded message, or the subject describes imagery which the subject then conjures up in his or her head has been used to aid ill persons understand their diseases. In some cases a "dialogue" is enacted between the patient and the imagery, the purpose being to gather information about the illness.

Several suggestions have been put forward for people who have difficulty in visualizing:

- Bridging. Some people have an area of sensory awareness that they prefer to use. The preferred state is used as an access to a visual image.

- Turning off verbal "noise." This is done by deliberately scanning the environment without categorizing, labeling, or naming what is seen. It is thought that when poor visualizers are deprived of words for what they see, they will resort to images.

- Visual recall with the use of a slide projector in which the item on the slide is allowed to be seen for only a very brief time

- Evoking visual images of something one strongly enjoys looking at

- Evoking early childhood memories

- Dream recall

- Picturing inner dialogues as cartoons[15]

Visualization has been used in autogenic training, biofeedback, and hyponosis, as discussed here, and in several forms of meditation. In the latter case it has been found to alter electroencephalographic brain wave patterns[16] and psychophysiology.[17-20] Since there is this intimate connectivity among the mind, psychological processes, and the physical body as an integrated system, a potent therapy has been developed for selected persons with cancer by the Simontons and Creighton.[21] Their method combines the use of visualization to promote psychological awareness and self-care with the standard medical treatment of chemotherapy and radiation. This highly successful therapy gives the patients an opportunity to actively participate in their own health care by learning to relax to break the recycling of uncontrollable fear and rising tensions that are the common lot of those who are told "There is nothing more that medical science can do . . . " This they do by unstressing their bodies through relaxation techniques and by using positive affirmation and guided imagery in a manner that will charge them with an expectant attitude toward meeting short-term goals in their quest for wellness. This program is carried out with the guidance of a counseler who cares about the inidividual and the resources of an "Inner Guide" who also is invoked through imagery.

The theoretical foundation for the relationship between physical disease, in this case cancer, and the cognitive processes involved in imagery is based on three known factors. One of these bases is the surveillance theory as developed by Prehn. In this theory the success of abnormal cells to break through the body's immune system is rare and, therefore, abnormal cells, such as cancer cells, are seen as being vulnerable to attack from the immune system. In addition, cancer cells are considered "metabolically confused" and open to this attack. Another basis is the extensive literature on the relationship between stress and the development of cancer and other diseases.[22] The works of both Riley[23] and Solomon and Amkraut[24] demonstrate that unrelieved stress significantly weakens the immune system by altering crucial hormone levels. The third component in the theoretical frame of reference is concerned with principles of biofeedback (see above) by which persons can learn to consciously control functions of the autonomic nervous system.

Achterberg and Lawlis developed a unique psychological instrument, the IMAGE-CA, to draw out from patients undergoing imagery therapy discussion about their imagery drawings.[25] This standardized instrument has provided a communication link between therapist and patient and it engages the patient in his or her own therapeutic process. On the basis of the psycological variables that are evoked by the instrument, it enables the team of therapists to anticipate the course of the patient's disease process as this can be elicited through the reflection of the state of the patient's coping mechanisms that can be deduced through the IMAGE-CA testing results.

Meditation

Essentially there are two phases to meditation: (1) centering or coming into relationship with self and (2) the perceiving in quietude how mind, or consciousness, works. In the words of the Quaker writer Bradford Smith, it is an "inward art" the essence of which each person must capture for himself or herself.

As noted above, several studies have demonstrated that it is possible to significantly alter psychophysiologic responses through meditative practices. Meditation is a worldwide practice of ancient origin (see particularly Chap. 4). In most ages meditation has been practiced within a religious context. However, as a holistic health practice in our age this has not necessarily been the case. Meditation as practiced today is more eclectic, drawing from many techniques. Basically what is sought is a shift in consciousness, for sensitivity is too frequently downgraded by routine acts of daily living in the present technology-bound world. Through meditative practice increasing sensitivity to subtle stimuli may occur. This can allow the meditator to refresh his or her powers of perception even in environments that are seemingly bleak and drab. An intimation of unity and wholeness can accompany developed meditative practice, giving one a sense of transpersonal experience and of deepened self-knowledge.[26]

One of the outcomes of meditation is a better understanding of the many facets of self and an appreciation for previously unperceived potentialities. As the meditative experience is translated into one's daily life, the perspective changes as these potentialities are explored and finally actualized. As the reality of the fullness of self is experienced, "... the practice of this approach leads to less vulnerability, greater inner freedom, less attachment to particular feeling states or opinions and therefore greater flexibility, all in the direction of mental health."[27]

A practical Westernized centering technique that closely resembles transcendental meditation, the Clinically Standardized Meditation, has been developed by Carrington.[28] As the name suggests, the method has been standardized and used clinically by psychotherapists in both hospitals and private practice.

Unlike in transcendental meditation (TM), trainees in the Clinically Standardized Meditation can either make up their own mantra in accordance with some simple rules provided by Carrington or they can select one from a pool of 16 Sanskrit mantras whose word-sounds have been validated by a panel of judges known to be experts in the yoga tradition of mantra meditation.

The mantra is the core of this centering technique. The practice is done in a quiet, pleasant atmosphere. The instructions for the centering process are purposely permissive, but the instructions themselves are standardized. The major regulation concerns the length of time the trainee does the technique, and this is regulated on an individual basis. The procedure is without religious context of any kind; however, "... a short, standardized, soothing means of transferring the mantra (which he or she has personally selected)" is done as a planned ritual to enhance the learning milieu.

In essence, the technique is concerned with the provision of a permissive, relaxing atmosphere in which one can feel free to allow the welling up of usually repressed facets of consciousness and to become quietly aware of the fullness of one's own stature.

Experiential Exercise

The purpose of this exercise is to help the individual experience ordering principles within his or her own psyche as a means of recognizing a unitary directing principle that is primary in the formation and sustenance of his or her own personal patterns of growth.

1. Work with a partner, preferably someone with whom you do not as yet have a strong acquaintance. Decide between you which one shall experience creative imagery first. The other person will play the role of a human support system to that person; that is, he or she will listen; will encourage verbalization without any attempt to be judgmental, analytical or coercive; will make notes; will quietly sit near his or her partner; and will begin by softly reading aloud the next section (2), below:

2. The person undergoing the experience should:

   a. Gently close the eyes and relax

   b. It may be useful to imagine a screen in front of your mind's eye and then allow yourself to quietly observe and describe the flow of imagery that moves across this screen.

   c. Try not to be self-conscious about this flow. Look upon the images that move across the screen in an objective manner as an observer of an interesting story. Do not attempt to structure the flow of images; just permit them to arise freely. Permit the imagery to speak to you.

   d. If you remember dream content, describe the dream to your support person, and while doing so, effortlessly drift back down into the dream so that you feel as though you are recapturing the feeling tone or the atmosphere of that dream.

   e. When you feel that you are again in that space, try to continue or extend that dream. Again, do not force structure upon the imaging; allow the images to flow as they will and describe them as they flow by the screen in your mind's eye.

3. At the end of the experience change roles.

4. When both partners have had their turn, discuss your experiences with each other and fill in any impressions of your experience that you could not articulate at the time you visualized them. Should further reminiscences or reflections arise to conscious awareness later in the week, add them also to this account, which can be kept in a continuing journal. During this time you may want to reexperience your dream and imaging. Do not force the material; allow your psyche to unfold its contents to your conscious awareness unimpeded by any willful structuring on your part. Allow it to reveal itself to you on its own terms, in accordance with its own internal rhythms. Allow it to teach you about yourself in a way only it can do. As with any committed teacher, material forthcoming will be most creative, clear, and cogent where the student is alert, enthusiastic, and eager for learning. Be it.

Summary

Only a few of the multitude of holistic health practices have been reviewed. It becomes apparent upon close examination that these practices loosely fall under either the category of a somewhat dissociative frame of mind as in autosuggestion or the category of conscious practice such as meditation. Most of the practices derive from transcultural, frequently ancient, sources. Some synthesize the transcultural with modern techniques and knowledges (*i.e.,* biofeedback). The common denominator is that the practice allows the individual to experience, and thereby become more aware of, self. This is done by an inward focusing and persistent search for subtle cues to latent facets of consciousness that can then be brought more fully into awareness and actualized.

References

1. Beals AR: Strategies of resort to curers in South India. In Leslie C (ed): Asian Medical Systems, pp 184–200. Berkeley, University of California Press, 1977
2. Sobel D: Introduction, ancient systems of medicine. In Sobel D (ed): Ways of Health: Holistic Approaches to Ancient and Contemporary Medicine, p 108. New York, Harcourt, Brace, & Jovanovich, 1979
3. Jung CG: Commentary. In Wilhelm R: The Secret of the Golden Flower, 2nd ed, p 83. London, Oxford University Press, 1962
4. Clement FE: Primitive Concepts of Disease. University of California Publications in American Archeology and Ethnology 32, No. 2, 1932
5. Durckheim KG: A practice to achieve man's wholeness. *Image* 64:3, 1974
6. Durckheim, *Loc cit*
7. Green E, Green A: The ins and the outs of mind-body energy. In Science Year, 1974, p 138. Chicago, Field Enterprises, 1973
8. Frankel F, Zamansky H (eds): Hypnosis and Its Bicentennial: Selected Papers. New York, Plenum, 1979
9. Hilgard E: Divided Consciousness. New York, John Wiley, 1978
10. Luthe W (ed): Autogenic Training. New York, Grune & Stratton, 1969
11. Miller NE, et al: Learned modification of autonomic functions. In Barber TX, et al (eds): Biofeedback and Self Control. Chicago, Aldine-Atherton, 1970
12. Green E, Green A, *op cit*, p 146
13. Biofeedback in Neuromuscular Reeducation. Biofeedback Research Institute, 6325 Wilshire Blvd., Los Angeles, 90048
14. Microcomputers revolutionizing biofeedback, Brain/Mind 4, No. 4:2, 1978
15. Exercises for sharpening vision in the mind's eye. Brain/Mind 4, No. 17:2, 1979
16. Kamiya J: Operant control of the EEG alpha rhythm and some of its reported effects on consciousness. In Tart CT (ed): Altered States of Consciousness, pp 507–517. New York, John Wiley & Sons, 1969

17. Brosse T: A psychophysiological study. Main Currents in Modern Thought 4:77–84, 1946
18. Kasamatsu A, Hirai T: An EEG study on the zen meditation (Zazen). In Tart CT (ed): Altered States of Consciousness, pp 489–501. New York, John Wiley & Sons, 1969
19. Wallace RK: Physiological effects of transcendental meditation. Science 167:1751–1754, 1970
20. Wallace RK, Benson H: The physiology of meditation. Sci Am 226:84–90, 1972
21. Simonton OC, Matthews-Simonton S, Creighton J: Getting Well Again. Los Angeles, JP Tarcher, 1978
22. Achterberg J, Simonton OC, Matthews-Simonton S: Stress, Psychological Factors and Cancer: an Annotated Bibliography. Fort Worth, New Medicine Press, 1976
23. Riley V: Mouse mammary tumors: alteration of incidence as apparent function of stress. Science 189:465–467, 1975)
24. Solomon GF, Amkraut AA: Emotion, stress and immunity. Frontiers of Radiation Therapeutic Oncology 1:84–96, 1972
25. Achterberg J, Lawlis GF: Imagery of Cancer. Champaigne, Institute for Personality and Ability Testing, 1978
26. Ornstein RE: The Psychology of Consciousness, pp 104–140. San Francisco, WH Freeman, 1972
27. Naranjo C: The One Quest, p 178. New York, Viking Press, 1972
28. Carrington P: Freedom in Meditation. New York, Anchor Books, 1978

7 Current Modalities in Holistic Health Practice

The range of holistic health practices is as varied as human beings are complex. Many of these practices are essentially similar but are called by different names. Frequently the difference is simply that two or more modalities arise from different ethnic sources, such as acupressure (Chinese) and *shiatsu* (Japanese), rather than from distinctly different techniques. The major reason at this time for a modality to be included among holistic health practices is that it adds to the practitioner's knowledge about himself or herself and therefore helps the person to actualize his or her potential for well-being. There are very few, if any, persons who have studied all of the available techniques affording access to the complexities of human nature. At the time of this writing, there have been no succinct articulation and classification of holistic health practices into integrated systems. Therefore, reflecting the obvious delimitations of the writer, the following account of holistic health practices restricts itself to about three dozen of those that are most popularly known. This is an acknowledged arbitrary basis for choice. The reason for summarizing these several modalities is to give the reader a basis to begin his or her own search for appropriate holistic health practices and to provide an overview of the possibilities for client referral. For purposes of convenience, the modalities are listed in alphabetical order under the broad generalizations of modalities concerned with (1) nonallopathic (*i.e.*, practices that are not disease-oriented) methods of diagnosis, (2) the rebalancing of human energies, (3) the relationship of body structure to environmental forces, and (4) awareness of self.

Nonallopathic Diagnostic Modalities

Applied Kinesiology

The innovative feature that applied kinesiology brings into focus is the translation of the body language exhibited by the client into diagnostic cues. The rationale underlying this mode of diagnosis is that there is a clear correlation between the ways people position their bodies, which reflect muscular weaknesses and consequent structural imbalance, and the state of their viscera. In fact, the muscle weakness represents motoneuron inhibitions and these inobtrusively pattern body language and can reflect fundamental visceral problems.

The tool by which this language is read is muscle testing of various reflex centers in the body. These centers are based on composite studies of neurovascular reflexes, neurolymphatic reflexes, and acupuncture reflexes, which indicated that for a weakness or dysfunction of a particular organ, for instance the kidneys, there will be a concomitant demonstrable weakness in a specific muscle, for instance the psoas muscle. The relationship to the acupuncture reflex in the case cited is that the kidney meridian begins by proceeding from the sole of the front part of the foot and then the energy goes up the inner aspect of the lower leg and thigh to the bladder. These areas may be related functionally to the psoas major and the psoas minor muscles. It should perhaps be noted that the kidney meridian in its entirety goes beyond the bladder, in a physiologic sense, and travels upward (caudally) through the unbilical area and the sternum and ends on the sternal side of the clavicle. Goodheart, who was one of the earliest to structure and classify these kinds of relationships, states that similar relationships exist for foot reflexes, hand reflexes, areas in the eye that are concerned with iridology diagnostics (see later), and cranial reflex centers.[1]

A remarkable finding of applied kinesiology is called *therapy localization*, in which the hands of the client can act as the localizer or diagnostic tool to elicit the area of involvement. This is done by having the client place his or her hand in contact with the involved muscle area. If the reflex center is irritated or the function is altered in any way, and muscle testing is done at the same time as the client places his or her hands on the area, there is a reversal in the condition of that muscle: if it was weak before, it will now test out strong; if the muscle tested strongly before, it will now be weak as long as the client's hand remains on the involved area. These are empirical findings; at present there is no substantive theory for their occurrence. It is claimed that therapy localization coupled with other applied kinesiology techniques can diagnose, with few exceptions, all dysfunctions that have an effect on the nervous system.[2]

Iridology

In the last quarter of the nineteenth century, a minister in Sweden, N. Liljequist, and a medical doctor in Hungary, I. von Peczely, simultaneously became aware that the effects of disease, drugs, and chemicals on the physical body can be diagnosed from changes in the coloration and structure of the eye. Neither knew of the work of the other. In a tradition that goes back to the works of Liljequist and von Peczely, the underlying assumption of this art, *iridology*, is that every organ in the body has a representation area in the eye. In effect, the umbilical zone is assigned to the area of the eye surrounding the pupil, the abdomen and its contents encircle that area, and then regions radiate out to the periphery of the eye, each radiation represeting one of the other organs and key structures of the body. A schema of different colorations is assigned to four major classifications of pathology: (1) acute inflammatory conditions, (2) subacute inflammation, (3) chronic conditions, and (4) destruction of tissues. Isolated pigmentation of various areas in the iris indicates mineral or drug deposits in the corresponding part of the body.

It is claimed that symptoms of pathology and the general state of the body's health are reflected in the condition of the iris, and this is the basis or iridologic diagnosis. Because of the sensitivity of these tissues to biochemical changes in the body, particularly those caused by toxicity or autonomic nervous system changes, the patient's progress in treatment can be closely monitored or a change in condition can be known well before there are physical manifestations apparent in the rest of the body.[3]

Psychic Readings

Shamanic practices (see Chap. 2) suggest that the use of psychic readings for diagnostic and prognostic purposes extends back into the far reaches of human history. In modern times the most famous psychic reader was Edgar Cayce, who in professional life was a photographer.[4] Cayce's career as a pscychic reader began when, at about the age of 21, it was noticed that he was developing a gradual paralysis of his throat muscles. Repeated medical examinations failed to find any physical cause for the progressive paralysis and finally hypnosis was tried, but without success.

Cayce had been a psychically perceptive child and, remembering that in his childhood he could obtain information from his unconscious during sleep, he solicited the help of a friend to put him into a hypnotic sleep by suggestion. Cayce was able to go into trance through his friend's suggestions and discern the basis of his paralysis. In his trance he was able to converse with his friend and allow material to well up from his unconscious without censoring it. In this way he was able to suggest medication and manipulative treatment for his throat, although later, when awake, he was not aware of how he did it. His throat condition soon healed.

Because of contingencies within his family and among his friends and neighbors, Cayce continued this mode of discerning the causes of illnesses and their treatment. A group of physicians in his hometown and in its outlying areas used Cayce's ability to diagnose their own patients' illnesses. It was found that once he was in trance and simply given the names and addresses of the patients under consideration, Cayce could telepathically obtain correct information about each patient and then could go on to diagnose the patient's condition and suggest treatment. When he was awake, however, he was not at all aware of these experiences. The verity of his information and the validity of his suggested treatments were demonstrated with unusual frequency, and finally his fame grew beyond the confines of his hometown Hopkinsville, Kentucky and eventually reached worldwide proportions.

For 43 years, Cayce regularly did these trance sessions, and a collection of 14,246 statements accrued that had been taken down by a stenographer during Cayce's trances. Of these psychic readings, it is said that 8,976 were descriptions of illnesses and suggestions for their treatments.[5]

One of the treatments most frequently suggested by Cayce was the application of castor oil packs.[6] McGarey has studied the known empirical effects of these packs but is unable to offer substantive theory for their effects. The castor oil pack consists of a piece of cotton material that has been soaked in castor oil (*Racinus communis*), and for treatment purposes the pack is placed externally over the locality of the body that is affected. Its cleansing and detoxifying effects are said by McGarey to work through the lymphatics that are stimulated by the pack.

Persons having the ability to do psychic readings have been intensively studied in this century. Although much evidence for the validity of the phenomenon has accrued both through personal accounts[7] and formal psychoanalysis,[8] at the present time there is little scientifically acceptable theory to substantiate this extraordinary medium of communications. A fuller appreciation and understanding may rest not so much in the accumulation of more data as in an enlightened shift in our cultural mores.

Bioenergetic Analyzers

Psionics had its beginnings in a field representative of a new class of technology that has been the hallmark of the twentieth century: electricity and electronics. The precursor of psionics was *radionics*, a term introduced into the English language in the mid 1930s. Bioenergetic instrumentation developed under this aegis act as detectors of disease in humans, animals, and plants. The basis for the validity of these instruments is that they help to focus the practitioner's attention. However, to date it is not known how this happens, and presently the question that provokes the interest of investigators in the field of bioenergetics is whether the person working the instrument is an integral part of the detector circuitry.

The person best known for his early work in the field of bioenergetics was Albert Abrams, an unusually perceptive medical doctor who went on to do postdoctoral studies in physics under von Helmholz. His particular interest was in integrating biologic laws with the laws of physics.

Initially, Abrams' interest was aroused when he noted that when he percussed a patient's abdomen during medical examination, there seemed to be a dull sound over specific areas of the abdomen and that these areas related in a one-to-one fashion with specific diseases. Trying to magnify the response, Abrams introduced into the process a variable resistance instrument. In time he found that samples of diseased blood placed on the machine could be assigned values measured in ohms when the resistance was varied, and that in this way he could come up with a diagnosis of the disease affecting the person from whom the sample was taken by referring to the measurement in ohms alone.[9]

Abrams carried this idea one step further to treat the disease. He connected the patient by wires and electrodes in circuit to the resistance box which had been turned to the readout in ohm values of the patient's disease. Abrams called this instrument an *oscilloclast*, and he treated the patient by transmitting a series of intermittent negative potentials and radio frequencies through the oscilloclast.

The oscilloclast was modified after Abrams' death, the initial modification being a rubber detector plate that replaced the percussion of the patient's abdomen. When this plate was stroked with the fingers, a noticeable tactile resistance was felt when the appropriate disease was tuned in. The resistances and inductances were also discarded and replaced with a series of dials. These were said to be able to "tune in on patients" even at a distance.

In a later version of the oscilloclast, vacuum tubes and condensers were used instead of resistances to tune into a client's disease. Perfected and patented by one of the early pioneers of radio and a Fellow in the Society of Electrical Engineers, Thomas G. Hieronymous, the detection instrument included a radio frequency amplifier, variable condensers, and a noninductive resistance focused through a crystal prism. The rubber induction plate was retained for diagnostic purposes.

With the publication of Hieronymous' patent in 1949, the instrument was variously duplicated and tested. Eventually, however, it was recognized that the underlying basis of the Hieronymous instrument was not its design, but rather that the device merely helped the practitioner to focus concentration on the patient and on the diagnosis. The startling suggestion accepted in many quarters today is that in some still undetermined way the practitioner uses his or her own bodily state as a context or reference for diagnosis and that the instrument itself allows the practitioner to engage in this interiorized analysis. This conjecture has since gained some credence through the successful substitution of a symbolic representation of the instrument, for instance a diagram, for the actual nuts-and-bolts instrument itself.

Nevertheless, the diagnostic and treatment instruments were meticulously standardized by De la Waar in England. After repeated trials at his laboratories, it was found that about 30% of people who would lend themselves to training with the instrument could become successful diagnosticians. The crucial characteristics seem to be an unbiased mind, an ability for clear visualization, a willingness to build up considerable experience with the use of the instrument, and a foundation in medical knowledge. These are essentially the same characteristics that have always been required over time for this ancient practice, which is essentially based on techniques of dowsing. In its more recent practice, psionics has been coupled with Eastern knowledge on acupuncture points (see Chap. 3) and *cakras* (see Chap. 4).[10]

Methods of Rebalancing Energy

Acupuncture and Acupressure

The theory underlying acupuncture is discussed in Chapter 3, the Chinese Sphere of Influence. The Chinese traditional conception of health is intrinsically related to Chinese philosophy. Essentially, Chinese thought is based on the macrocosm–microcosm principle in that the natural laws of the universe are reflected in the laws that govern the well-being of man. As life energy, *ch'i*, continuously flows through the universe so too does *ch'i* constantly flow through and energize humans. This flow in humans occurs through particular conduits, called *meridians*, within which lies a series of localizations, called *acupoints*, through which *ch'i* may be intercepted.

Stimulation or sedation of the flow of *ch'i* is indicated, dependent upon a constellation of factors. These include whether the situation to be rebalanced is *yin* or *yang* or a combination of both, the person's nutritional state, and so on (see Orbisiconography, Chap. 3). If the flow of *ch'i* is impeded through either environmental factors or internal problems, either a build-up or a deficit of *ch'i* may result. Sedation in the first instance or stimulation in the second instance can be accomplished through the insertion of very fine needles into the acupoints. These needles are then twirled in a specific manner. The purpose of the twirling is to mechanically simulate the action of *ch'i*.

Twirling, which has traditionally been done by the rapid manipulation of the needle between the fingers, has more recently been supplanted or assisted by stimulation through electricity, ultrasound, and laser beam.

All acupoints except those around the eyes, ears, and large blood vessels may be treated by acupuncture. In these exceptional cases, however, a type of massage called *acupressure* is preferred. In general, acupressure uses a deep-pressure massage at the sites of the acupoints, the treatment being done with these of the index finger, the middle finger, or the positioning of the middle finger on the index finger to add forcefully to the pressure.[11] In acupressure therapy all of the acupoints are used as needed. A synthesis of oriental and occidental techniques, called *G-Jo*, has developed for self-help, particularly in the case of first aid. This finger-pressure technique has been particularly oriented toward paramedical use.[12]

Aikido

Aikido means pathway or road (*do*) to identification or union (*ai*) with the life energy (*ki*) that flows throughout the universe. It is a dyadic interaction in which the basic principle is one of nonresistance. Extreme sensitivity to one's opponent allows one to be constantly aware of the intended movements of the opponent. The underlying thrust of the teaching is to learn to be in a position that allows one to use the opponent's momentum against the opponent.

Aikido movements are the microcosm of the universe's macrocosmic movements. The teaching of *Aikido* stresses the importance of allowing one's self to move with change, openly and with a sense of the order which governs the microcosm as it does the macrocosm. To do this one must learn to find one's center and thereby quiet the mind, balance the body, and seek out one's spiritual relationship to the universe and all life in it.[13]

The major center of the body is the solar plexus *cakra*, called *hara* in Japanese. As noted in Chapter 4, the *cakras* are nonphysiologic centers for energy input. Through their controlled use the student learns to uncover universal laws and to live naturally and harmoniously with them in everyday life, for the essence of *Aikido* is to experience and thereby know that there is a direct correspondence between *hara*, the body's center, and the center of the universe. Their active cultivation gives one immovable power and integration of body, mind, and spirit.

Aikido was originally taught as a martial art to adults and was also adopted as a form of therapy in which a person confronts his or her own aggression. However, one of the best uses I have ever seen it put to was in the treatment of hyperkinetic children. Through the use of *Aikido* these children learned for the first time that they need not automatically respond to the uncontrolled movements of their body, but that through the use of mental alertness, intentionality, and balance they could ground their bodies and move them as they willed.

Chiropractic

Chiropractic was founded by D. D. Palmer in the closing days of the nineteenth century. The basic principles of chiropractic are concerned with the maintenance of the structural and functional integrity of the nervous system. The methods used in its practice are primarily those of manipulation and adjustment of joints and the underlying tissues, and are based on the natural curative abilities of the body itself. Because of this, chiropractic also supports programs of natural nutrition and recognizes the detrimental role of everyday stress in modern life-styles. The major mode of treatment is directed toward the neuromechanic and kinesiologic features which cause spinal and pelvic misalignments, problems of radiating pain due to interference with spinal nerve conduction, general muscular ailments, and visceral dysfunctions due to compression or mechanical irritation of nerves.[14] A major breakthrough in chiropractics occurred with the teaching of applied kinesiology by Goodheart (see above) through which weakened muscles and nerves can be readily diagnosed.

Homeopathy

Homeopathy was founded by Samuel Hahneman in the early nineteenth century. Its basic tenet is the Principle of Similars, which states that (1) the normally healthy body is dependent on an ability to maintain balance of its energies; (2) the body's basic pattern of health is the determinant of recovery from illness; (3) most symptoms of illness are holistic, encompassing the physical, emotional, and mental aspects of the individual; and (4) when medication is given to a healthy person systematically, his or her symptoms will be specific. Based upon the latter assumption, patients are given extensive examinations so that their particular and individual symptoms are elicited. The individualized symptomatology is then closely matched to the prescribed remedy from a *materia medica* of more than one thousand medications, and the medication is given in the minimum effective dose. Perhaps this is the reason homeopathy has an acknowledged safety record with persons who are allergic or who have had severe drug reactions, and with children and persons in very weakened conditions.

Naturopathic Medicine

Naturopathy uses "nature's agencies, forces, processes, and products" in an attempt to maintain the natural physiology and normal biochemistry of the body. Its approach is multidisciplinary, in which botanical medicine, homeotherapeutics, physiotherapy, minor surgery, manipulation, and preventive medicine, as well as methods of prepared or natural childbirth, are used for the well-being of the patient. Therapies are eclectic and may include colon irrigations, supervised fasting, herbs, chelation, deep nerve massage, chiropractic manipulations, physiotherapy, hyperbaric oxygen treatment, and acupuncture. Naturopathic physicians treat all conditions of illness, ranging through the realm of the general allopathic physician. These include such diversity as cardiovascular, neurologic, orthopedic, musculoskeletal, gastrointestinal, genitourinary, pulmonary, and dermatologic problems in any age range.

Polarity Therapy

Polarity therapy in its present form was developed by Randolph Stone as a synthesis of Eastern and Western medicine and philosophy. It includes manipulation practices, contact with both hands on pressure-sensitive points throughout the body, a polarity yoga consisting of various stretching exercises, a diet that includes herbs, and studies of the flow and balance of energy in daily life.

Polarity therapy aims at the repatterning of energy flow in the individual by using that individual's own energy field. Essentially this occurs through the attraction of opposites, that is, positive and negative charges. Certain parts of the body are positive or negative to other parts of the body. The hands and fingers also have positive and negative charges. To balance energy, the practitioner places a finger or a whole hand on parts of the patient's body of opposite charge and thereby facilitates energy balancing where it is needed.[15]

Psychic Healing

Psychic healing is a very ancient mode of helping or healing ill people that goes back in recorded history to practice in Egyptian temples of healing. The term *psychic healing* is frequently used synonymously with *faith healing* and *spiritual healing,* largely because one aspect of psychic healing, the laying-on of hands, usually takes place within a religious context. Healing at a distance, another form of psychic healing, is done during meditation or prayer. Psychic healing is assumed to occur through the transference of a healing energy from the healer to the healee, the healer acting as a channel for this transference.[16]

Reflexology

The practice of reflexology is based on the assumption that over 72,000 nerves in the body terminate in the feet. It is further said that there are ten zones in the body and each zone has a corresponding area reflected on the soles of the feet. When there is a problem or disease in the body, the area on the feet that correlates with the zone of the body in which the problem manifests itself will become crystallized with deposits of calcium and acids. Therefore, treatment is directed toward breaking up these deposits. Once the condition is relieved, incipient imbalances of energy can then be treated before problems arise. Reflexology is also known as *zone therapy.*[17]

Therapeutic Touch

Therapeutic Touch will be described later in this chapter and in Part 3 of this book.

Relationship of Body Structure to Environmental Forces

The Alexander Technique

The Alexander Technique was developed by F. M. Alexander out of his own personal experience. Alexander was a Shakespearean actor in the late nineteenth century. He frequently lost the use of his voice, for which he sought several avenues of help, none of which were successful. Finally, aided by the positioning of several mirrors, he studied his body as he spoke. He realized that part of his problem was caused by the way he habitually held his body as he spoke. As he further studied his body he recognized that his body acted as a whole, that the problem with his voice was not one of isolated movement, but rather that the movement occurred as a result of the integration of several facets of his body, his personality, and his thought.

After many years Alexander returned to the theater, and those who had not seen him in some time were very impressed by the way he was able to use his breath. He began to teach other actors what he had learned from his own experiences. Central to his teaching was that learning the technique could not be an intellectual appreciation only; in order for the learning to be significant, there had to be a kinesthetic experience in which the concept was personally worked through.[18] To understand the proper use of self in relation to the environment, the student is encouraged in the practice of psychophysical ecology, the intelligent awareness of the interdependence of all facets of self in daily acts of living, and the synergistic effects of those acts on one's habitual life-style.[19]

Dance Therapy

Although dancing in groups is one of the most ancient of art forms, dance as a conjunct of psychotherapy is a new dance form, one of the few forms of psychotherapy that is American in origin. Its basic concepts are concerned with the use of rhythm to bind people together into a cohesive whole. In the freedom, sometimes abandon, of rhythmic sound and movement, the acting out of new roles and new interpretations of self is supported.

Dance as a healing art form came to popular attention through the work of Marion Chace, who was able to reach even grossly dissociated psychiatric patients through dance. By using dance to help patients to express their often inarticulate conflicts, pain, and body language, Chace was able to create an objective base for their self-awareness, a means for freely expressing this recognition, and a learning of how to integrate their behaviors in a permissive environment.[20] The dance therapist today is a clinician who has an integrated knowledge of the psychotherapeutic effects of group and individual movement.[21]

Feldenkrais Method

Moshe Feldenkrais, Ph.D., has a unique background as a physicist and as a black-belt expert in judo. His analytical mind plus his experience with body movement led him to the understanding that if the individual is intelligently taught about body functioning, that individual can give knowledgeable guidance to his or her body in daily life. By giving the individual gentle manipulations so that the awareness of the body increases, that person can make more informed choices about how to manipulate the body in space. Coupled with this is a philosophical base in which exploration of self is encouraged and responsibility for self is supported in the direction of constructive alteration of self-image and awareness of other.[22]

Lomi Body Work

Lomi body work is a method of psychophysical therapy that was developed by R. K. Hall, a physician, and R. K. Heckler, Ph.D. Introduced in 1971, the basic theory underlying this method is that an individual's character is expressed physically through the state of his or her awareness, vitality and vigor, breathing patterns, and structural balance. By directing attention to current muscular tension, an individual learns to restructure postural alignment so that there can be a free flow of body energies, and to integrate both emotional as well as physical energies in natural ways according to universal laws governing human energy flow.[23]

Rolfing

The founder and major developer of the Rolf System of Structural Integration was Ida P. Rolf, Ph.D. The practice, known as rolfing, is based on a theory that the body is not a unit, but rather an aggregate of large segments (*i.e.*, the head, the thorax, the pelvis, the legs). The body is seen as a plastic, movable medium of collagen structures that can alter its characteristics in direct relation to its energy level. In physiologic terms, this change runs the spectrum from the more compact or solid gel state to the looser or more fluid sol state.

The purpose of rolfing is to help the rolfee establish deep structural relationships within the body that express themselves through symmetrical and balanced functioning when the body is in an upright position. To provide visual feedback to the healees, both measurements and photographs of their bodies are taken for baseline reference and again during the course of the learning of structural integration. In structural integration the forces of the gravitation field are deliberately used so that the energy level of the body is enhanced. Emotional trauma may also be locked up in the body's habitual stance. Therefore, it is thought that the biochemical changes in the myofacia, which occur as a result of the manipulation of muscles as the body is aligned as an integrated and balanced energy system, serve to release emotion as well.[24]

Stress Reduction

Techniques of stress reduction will be discussed in Part 3 of this book.

Therapeutic Massage

Although literature on massage indicates that the use of massage goes back to the year 3000 B.C. among the Chinese, the word itself comes from the Greek *masso*, meaning I shape or knead (with the hands). In massage, in addition to kneading, there is (1) stimulation of muscle groups by a variety of methods such as stroking, pinching, vibration, shaking, and striking in a controlled manner, (2) *shiatsu*, a finger-pressure method of massage of acupoints, or (3) *ammo*, an oriental method of stimulating nerves which produce organic dysfunction.[25] The importance of therapeutic massage is to help make the client aware of the body's daily interaction with the environment and the areas of tension that build up inobtrusively.[26]

Awareness of Self

Art Therapy

Art therapy is an expressive modality characterized by the use of symbolic communication presented in any of the art media. The goal is to invoke spontaneous artistic creativity which will help the individual to break out of the self-made barriers of psychologic defense structures. With the help of the therapist, the client interprets his or her art creations from a symbolic perspective. This may lead to increased self-awareness, recognition of the roots of conflict and frustration, and the acknowledgment of repressed emotions.

Art therapy is very effective with persons who are unable to verbalize their problems, such as patients who are brain damaged, deeply depressed, hysteric, and so on. Art therapy can relate to all psychologic frames of reference. In the humanistic approach developed by Garai, the therapeutic goal is oriented toward reinforcing the will to live and toward supporting endeavors to find meaning and identity in as fully a creative life-style as is possible. Acceptance of inevitable change is fostered, and, in this context, clients' identity crises are redirected into creative–expressive life-styles where further experiences of change are expected and accepted. A spiritual framework in which to seek meaning for life is accepted and self-transcendent goals are supported.[27]

Drama Therapy

As art therapy uses spontaneous art for projective purposes, drama therapy uses spontaneous enactment through improvisation, role-playing, dramatic games, and creative drama, or specific clinical techniques.

Although the idea of drama therapy arose among various writers of the nineteenth century, in this country it is through psychodrama and sociodrama as conceived by Moreno that drama therapy is best known.[28] All modes of self-expression are used, but all are expressioned through modes of improvisation. Drama therapy is used with physically and psychologically disabled people, the retarded, the aged, and the deprived.[29]

Gestalt Therapy

The person who developed gestalt therapy to its most definitive form is Fritz Perls. The attempt in gestalt therapy is to perceive experience within the context of the whole, but from where one is existentially. The configuration of life experience is so integrated into the time and space of the individual—through memories in reference to events of the past and through anticipation concerning events yet to be perceived— that the therapeutic thrust is toward whatever is presently available to the client and the therapist and can be shared at the present moment. Therefore, this existential frame of reference allows both therapist and client to use whatever resources are accessible to either or both of them. Because any appropriate modalities to which the therapist has access may be used within the gestalt framework, the therapeutic relationship is made into a continuing innovative experience. Thus all of the therapies discussed in this chapter may be integrated into the therapeutic sessions, the type of modality used being dependent only on the therapeutic style of the gestalt therapist.[30]

Humanistic Psychology

Humanistic psychology has several sources; however, the seminal concept of self-actualization was the brainchild of Kurt Goldstein, a physician. Working with brain-injured patients, Goldstein was surprised and impressed by his patients' drive toward growth despite their devastating disabilities. The intensity of this drive was such that it enabled the patients to achieve a state of well-being far beyond what would have been predictable on the basis of medical evidence alone. This demanded a reinterpretation of the scope of human potentialities and laid the foundation for what was to become known as humanistic psychology.

Further work under Abraham Maslow added exploratory findings to the known range of human capacity.[31] Concomitantly, studies in the alternative therapies of biofeedback and self-control and healing and meditation, as well as the rise of the concept of responsibility for self, have filled the literature with specific instances of the power of self-actualization in the service of the ego.

Jungian Psychology

The core of humanistic psychology is holistic, and its thrust is toward the respect and support of the entire spectrum of being.[32] This interpretation of the psychologic nature of man rests on the work of Carl Gustav Jung. Jung realized the potency of expression of one's spiritual nature and recognized that the full articulation of this aspect of human life is cloaked in symbols. Underlying the fundamental symbolic expressions of one's life, which are merely glimpsed in dreams, fantasy, myth, and art, is a realm of unconscious energies that have not as yet been bound in thought. The binding of these energies awaits the catalyst provided by awareness to make them accessible to consciousness. Therefore, an important aspect of Jungian psychology is concerned with the clarification of symbolic imagery and the release of unconscious content.[33]

Psychosynthesis

Roberto Assegoli, an Italian psychiatrist, was the founder of the practice of psychosynthesis. Psychosynthesis is concerned with a conscious synthesis and unification of all facets of the self, the whole person. It is not only concerned with freedom from personal trauma and sorrow but also with experiencing the higher, transpersonal consciousness, in order to release through that self the unifying energies of universal Love, Joy, Beauty, Courage, and Wisdom. This transpersonal experience is marred by identification with subpersonalities, such as the Victim or Martyr within, or the Fearful Child, the Visionary Seeker, the Compulsive Helper, the Critical Judge, and so on. The overriding aim of psychosynthesis is to bring the subpersonalities to conscious awareness so that the individual is not passively controlled by them. Various methods are used to do this: guided imagery, movement, gestalt therapy, dream work, creative imagery, meditation, journal keeping, symbolic art work, the development of the intuition, and so on.[34]

Transpersonal Psychology

Beyond the domains of psychoanalysis, behaviorism, and humanistic psychology lies a "fourth force in psychology": the realm of transpersonal psychology. Transpersonal psychology is a synthesis of Eastern wisdom and Western scientific findings on human consciousness. Present studies in transpersonal psychology include investigations of transpersonal experiences (*i.e.*, experiences which go beyond the ordinary ego boundaries and the usual limitations of space and time), meditation, biofeedback, psychic phenomena, various states of consciousness, healing, energy transformation, and body disciplines. Applications to education and to psychotherapy have been reported. The purpose of these studies is directed toward enlarging the current conceptions of health and wholeness and learning how to live within that larger vision.[35]

References

1. Goodheart GJ: Applied Kinesiology Research Manuals. Detroit, International College of Applied Kinesiology, 1964–1971
2. Goodheart GB, Schmitt WH: Applied kinesiology. In Kaslof LJ (ed):

Wholistic Dimensions of Healing: a Resource Guide, p 78. New York, Doubleday, 1978

3. Jensen B: Science and Practice of Iridology. Privately Published, Route #1, Box 52, Escondido, CA, 92025, *n.d.*

4. Stearn J: Edgar Cayce, the Sleeping Prophet. New York, Doubleday, 1968

5. Reilly HJ, Brod RH: The Edgar Cayce Handbook for Health Through Drugless Therapy, p xiv. New York, Macmillan, 1975

6. MacGarey WA: Edgar Cayce and the Palma Cristi. Edgar Cayce Foundation Medical Research Bulletin, Virginia Beach, Edgar Cayce Foundation, *n.d.*

7. Garrett EJ: Many Voices: the Autobiography of a Medium. New York, GP Putnam's Sons, 1968

8. Progoff I: The Image of An Oracle. New York, Garrett Publications, 1964

9. Russell EW: Report on Radionics—Science of the Future. London, Neville Spearman, 1973

10. Tansley DV: Radionics and the Subtle Anatomy of Man. London, Health Science Press, 1971

11. Houston FM: The Healing Benefits of Acupuncture, p 16. New Canaan, Keats, 1974

12. Blake M: The G-Jo Handbook. Davis, Falkynor Books, 1976

13. Tohei: Aikido in Daily Life. New York, Japan Publications, 1966

14. Dintenfass J: Chiropractic today. In Kaslof LJ (ed): Wholistic Dimensions in Healing: a Resource Guide, p 64. New York, Doubleday, 1978

15. Stone R: Energy—the Vital Energy in the Healing Art. Published by Pierre Pannetier, Polarity Therapy, 401 North Glassell St., Orange, CA 92666, *n.d.*

16. Worrall AA, Worrall ON: The Gift of Healing. New York, Harper & Row, 1965

17. Fitzgerald WH, Bowers EF: Zone Therapy. Columbus, Ohio, IW Long, 1917

18. Alexander FM: The Use of Self. New York, EP Dutton, 1941

19. Tinbegan N: Ethology and stress diseases. Science pp 20–27, 1974

20. Chaikin H (ed): Marion Chace: Her Papers. Columbus, MD, American Dance Therapy Association, 1975

21. Pesso A: Movement in Psychotherapy. New York, New York University Press, 1969

22. Feldenkrais M: Awareness Through Movement. New York, Harper & Row, 1972

23. The Lomi Papers, Vols. I and II. Mill Valley, CA, Lomi School Press, 1975–1977

24. Rolf IP: Rolfing: the Integration of Human Structure. Santa Monica, Dennis-Landman, 1977

25. Katsusuke S: Massage: the Oriental Method. New York, Japan Publications, 1972

26. Downing G: The Massage Book. New York, Random House, 1972

27. Garai JE: Art Therapy: Catalyst for Creative Expression and Personality Integration. Englewood Cliffs, Prentice-Hall, 1977

28. Moreno JL: Psychodrama, Vols. I and II. New York, Beacon, 1959

29. Brown GI: Reach, Touch and Teach. New York, Viking Press, 1971

30. Perls F, Hefferline RF, Goodman P: Gestalt Therapy. New York, Dell, 1965

31. Maslow A: Toward a Psychology of Being. New York, VanNostrand Reinhold, 1968

32. Sutich A, Vich MA (eds): Readings in Humanistic Psychology. New York, Free Press, 1969
33. Singer J: Boundaries of the Soul. New York, Anchor Books, 1973
34. Assagoli R: Psychosynthesis: a Manual of Principles and Techniques. New York, Hobbs-Dorman, 1965
35. Keyes K: Handbook to Higher Consciousness. Berkeley, Living Love Center, 1975

8 Holism as a Conceptual Base of Professional Health Practices

Nursing, although it is one of the oldest avenues of human nurturing, has been very late in acknowledging that the vital conceptual basis for its growing body of theoretical knowledge must be, of necessity, holistic in nature. This necessity derives from the fact that the appropriate focus of nursing, both historically and currently, is human beings and the full stature of human beings can only be considered as a coherent whole, as a unified process.

Part of the reason for nursing's delay in acknowledging holism as the basis of its theoretical knowledge in modern times has been the strict adherence to an allopathic medical model within nursing education, nursing practice, and nursing research. This handmaiden-to-the-physician orientation in nursing developed as a historical error, a holdover from the early days of the twentieth century before either nursing or medicine had developed adequate theoretical content and before they had structured their unique services to society to qualify as *bona fide* professions.[1] It has been only comparatively recently that the medical model has been acknowledged to be invalid for professional nursing and that the way has been prepared for the lucid development of the body of knowledge that uniquely expresses nursing theory and clearly differentiates it from other professional disciplines.[2]

As the growing base of nursing theory has been developing, there has also been a concomitant recognition that creative and holistic alternatives for helping or healing people rightfully lie at the heart of professional nursing. These alternatives can constitute appropriate extensions of innovative nursing skills in clinical practice, research, and the development of the theory that underlies nurse education.[3]

The Rogerian Conceptual Model of Unitary Man

It was Martha E. Rogers' astute observation of nurses and nursing during the early 1960s that broke through the tradition-bound view of nursing as an intrinsic part of allopathic medicine. Rogers' perceptive and cogent analysis clarified the uniqueness of nursing: that the care of *people* is nursing's center of concern. Therefore, the singular appropriate context for nurse education is the study of generic man.

Rogers' conception of human beings is unitary. The human being is a holistic process, ". . . a synergistic phenomenon whose behaviors cannot be predicted by the parts," because the whole is, indeed, not only greater than the sum of the parts, but different. Rogers wrote as follows:

> The unity of man is a reality. Man interacts with his environment in his totality. Only as man's wholeness is perceived does the study of man begin to yield meaningful concepts and theories. Only as man's oneness is apprehended is it possible to identify man's distinctive attributes.[4]

Basic Assumptions of the Rogerian Model

The major premise of Rogers' model is that the universe is one of open systems (see Prigogine's theory of dissipative structures, Chap. 1) in which generic man and the environment coalesce as energy force fields. In that fusion, man and the environment are coextensive with the universe. This position posits a very human orientation: all there is within this universe of discourse is man and environment.

Noting that ". . . nursing theory is rooted in the broad foundation of knowledge that characterizes the liberally educated man,"[5] and that nursing shares this knowledge with other disciplines, Rogers proceeded to systematically organize and then synthesize, within the context of the wholeness of man and environment, concepts at the leading edge of knowledge about biologic, physical, and psychosocial human beings and their environment. Out of this synthesis a new thesis was developed, one with a theoretical base derived by inductive and deductive reasoning which sought to decisively differentiate nursing from other professional disciplines by virtue of a unique content of nursing knowledge. This growing body of new knowledge endeavors to explain the life process in humans and to describe their interaction with the universe. Thus, it attempts to provide an operational base for planned nursing interventions, the results of which can be predicted by the knowledgeable nurse.

There are five further basic assumptions underlying Rogers' conceptual model. To document the major biologic, physical, and psychosocial literature from which the cognative basis of this conceptual system logically derived, the appropriate references are provided in the parentheses after each of these five assumptions.

1. Man is a unified whole possessing his own integrity and manifesting characteristics that are more than and different from the sum of his parts.[6] (See references 7–16.)
2. Man and environment are continually exchanging matter and energy with one another.[17] (See references 18–27.)
3. The life process evolves irreversibly and unidirectionally along the space–time continuum.[28] (See references 29–37.)
4. Pattern and organization identify man and reflect his innovative wholeness.[38] (See references 39–49.)
5. Man is characterized by the capacity for abstraction and imagery, language and thought, sensation and emotion.[50] (See references 51–57.)

In addition to the above, Rogers specifies a pool of over 100 sources of significant related literature which she used for documentation of her thesis.[58]

The Rogerian Theoretical Base

The following assumptions are the context of the Rogerian conceptual system: man embodies a wholeness that cannot be appropriately understood from any one particular perspective. He is incessantly interacting with the environment through a time which is singularly future-oriented. Thus man is coupled with his surroundings in a nonstop dance of complementarity toward infinity. In this continuum each of the dancing partners changes and is changed by the other with a pattern and organization that are themselves characterized by that change. This pattern and organization are, therefore, emergent, unprecedented, and ever innovative. Because of this incessant becoming, unitary man cannot be understood by considerations that are anything less than holistic. Indications of his unitary nature, however, can be inferred from his unique characteristics for abstraction and imagery, language and thought, sensation and emotion.

Within this context, man and environment are energy fields, each of which maintains its own integrity in a universe of open systems. The characteristics of these energy fields are perceived through dynamic phenomena that are syntropic; that is, they exhibit a fundamental drive toward order. The matrices of the human field and the environmental field are each considered to be four-dimensional. However, this four-dimensionality is not to be construed within the definitions of either mathematics or psychology; rather, its interpretation is humanistic and its dynamics are relativistic.

Principles of Homeodynamics

Rogers has proposed two general principles within the context of her conceptual system: (1) the principle of helicy and (2) the principle of resonancy. There is a third proposition, called the principle of complementarity, that may be subsumed under the principle of helicy. Rogers' principles of homeodynamics are stated as follows:

Principle of Helicy

The nature and direction of human and environmental change are continuously innovative and probabilistic. They are characterized by increasing diversity of human field and environmental field pattern and organization that emerge from the continuous, mutual, and simultaneous interaction between the human and environmental fields and that manifest nonrepeating rhythmicities.

Principle of Resonancy

The human field and the environmental field are identified by wave pattern and organization manifesting continuous change from lower-frequency, longer-wave patterns to higher-frequency, shorter-wave patterns.

Principle of Complementarity

There is a continuous, mutual, and simultaneous interaction process between human and environmental fields.

Suggestive Hypotheses and Theories

Rogers' broad generalizations provide a basis for further hypotheses concerning the general character and tendencies inherent in the development of unitary man. For instance, Rogers hypothesizes the flow of incessant change, which she proposes in her principle of complementarity, to be in the direction of "higher wave frequency field pattern and organization" which is characterized by "increasing diversity." Translated in human terms, this suggests to her a theory of accelerated evolution. At the forefront of this accelerated evolution are children currently thought to be hyperactive and adults with higher-wave-frequency vital signs, such as elevated blood pressure readings. Should further research substantiate these suggested theories, a new relative scaling of expected human norms must be devised, Rogers notes. Under such circumstances, the context of nursing practices of the future would be individual-oriented and open-ended so that the principles underlying the care given to that individual would be based on the existential state of his or her becoming and would be ever subject to change within the perspective of the best interests of the client.

The Rogerian Conceptual System as a Basis for Explaining Field Behaviors of Unitary Man

Rogers' conceptual system provides a model within the context of which descriptive, theoretical, and predictive principles or axioms can be tested through formal research processes. Rogers suggests several ideas, the validity of which can be authenticated by such modeling:

Paranormal Events

Rogers' conception of a four-dimensional human field is relativistic; that is, the time–space corridor of perception is, so to speak, tilted in the uniquely personal direction of each individual's perspective. Because this is so, Rogers indicates that there is a valid base for the reality of certain psychic phenomena, such as precognition and telepathy, because the "now" experience, or the present, for one individual is only relative to that individual, but may logically represent a quite different phasing of time to another person.

Human Field Rhythms

Within Rogers' frame of reference the rhythmicities so characteristic of human behavior are seen to be resultants of the holistic nature of the human field in mutual and simultaneous interaction with the environmental field and in consonance with the principle of helicy noted above. Research on indices of this human field motion is currently in process.

The Aging Process

Within Rogers' model human aging is always in process on a continuum that proceeds from conception through the dying process. This is conceived as an innovative developmental process oriented toward a growing diversity of human field pattern and organization. According to Rogers, one of the indicants of this is that there is less need for protracted periods of sleep among the aged and that the patterned frequencies of the sleep/wake cycle themselves demonstrate greater variety. As support for her thesis that the vectoring of human evolution is in the direction of higher-wave-frequency field pattern and organization, Rogers cites evidence that indicates that as people age, the direction of change in their color preferences is in the predicted direction, toward the colors of higher-wave frequencies.

A Nursing Care Study Based on the Rogerian Conceptual System

The nursing science context of holism in which behavior is perceived as human field phenomena is directly applicable in the clinical nursing situation, as well as in nurse education and nursing research. An example of its applicability to nursing practice is presented here in the nursing care plan of a second-year student in nursing science, Djuna Wendruff, with her permission. It will be noted that the nursing care plan discusses the use of Therapeutic Touch as an extension of the professional skills of the nurse. Therapeutic Touch has not been discussed thus far in this book; however, considerable consideration will be given to Therapeutic Touch in the clinical papers in Part 3. Briefly, Therapeutic Touch was first described by the author in 1972.[59] It is an act of healing or helping which derives from the laying-on of hands. Unlike the laying-on of hands, Therapeutic Touch is not done within a religious context, nor is the healing or helping that occurs considered to be a function of the faith of the healer or the healee (patient). Another notable difference is that, whereas in the laying-on

Nursing Care Plan

Nursing Diagnosis	**Rationale**
1. Impersonal hospital environment is dysynchronous with the simultaneous highly personal state of the maternal field.	1. Ms. R exhibits readily identifiable needs for personal space. Her admission to the hospital brings her energy field into relationship with the energy field of the hospital. The hospital environment is crowded with strange, unfamiliar phenomena: unknown people with demands for unsought intimacy with her, and unexpected sounds, sights, smells, and sensations. Significant loss of personal space and the relationship of this loss to various behavioral manifestations exemplify the reciprocal nature of the human/environmental field interaction.
2. Inability to move about decreases client's ability to maximize her potential for health.	2. Studies have been conducted on the effects of motion upon the human energy field.[67] The withdrawal of the ability to be in motion has resonating effects on the energy and potentiality of the client's field.

of hands the ability to heal is considered to be the result of a special gift or calling, in Therapeutic Touch the ability to play the role of healer is considered to be a natural potential in people that can be actualized under the appropriate circumstances.[60]

Several studies have demonstrated that treatment by Therapeutic Touch significantly affects hemoglobin values, hematocrit ratios,[61] brain waves,[62] and state–anxiety,[63] and brings about a generalized relaxation response[64] in the person so treated. At this writing, two doctoral dissertations on Therapeutic Touch have been completed for the Ph.D. degree in research and theory development in nursing science. Several others are in preparation in nursing and also in other professions.[65, 66]

For the purposes of this nursing care plan presentation, the client will be referred to as Ms. R. She is 28 years old and slightly obese, but she has a youthful appearance. She is lying in a labor bed preparatory to the delivery of her child. The siderails of the bed are up, and the head of the bed is elevated at a 30-degree angle. The bed is beside a window overlooking Central Park, a very large park in New York City. Ms. R's husband is standing close beside her and appears very attentive. A fetal monitor is attached and in place, and its electronic beeping tone is clearly audible.

Diagnosis	Supporting Data	Conflicting Data
# 1	Client appears withdrawn. Does not initiate contact with structures in the environmental field. She appears embarrassed by some of the procedures she is subjected to.	Client has not requested any of the hospital personnel to leave the labor room.
# 2	Contractions are increasing in severity, but client is unable to move her body in response to them. Due to fetal monitor, Ms. R attempts to hold back her	Although inability to move about freely may reduce health potential on some levels, the labor bed with the siderails is for the client's safety. Fetal

Nursing Diagnosis	**Rationale**
	Not only is Ms. R confined to a narrow labor bed, but she is also further immobilized by the attachment of internal fetal monitor leads to the scalp of the fetus within her. This situation renders her incapable of motion synchronous with the inherent and natural forces of labor.
3. Client is unable to maximize energy of contraction.	3. Labor contractions are rhythmic phenomena that function as expressions of the reciprocal relationship between the maternal field and the fetus' field. At this moment in space/time, the forces of labor are dysynchronous with the energy field of Ms. R. She is unable to concentrate and use breathing techniques in order to relax the uterine muscles. During the contractions Ms. R frowns and grimaces. Her whole being appears to tighten in resistance against the natural forces of labor. This dysrhythmic experience is overwhelming to her and prevents her from organizing her field in such manner as to efficiently utilize the powerful energies bound to the labor experience.
4. Client is not perpetuating energy flow within own system.	4. As her energy level dissipates owing to the great pain, fear, and fatigue she experiences, Ms. R is no longer capable of efficiently utilizing her own available resources. She does not participate in her own care, but allows other people to take complete care of her, thereby relinquishing control over her own labor and delivery.
5. There is constriction of human energy field.	5. Variation in field boundaries is associated with growth and development. Birthing is a process in the growth and development of women. In a crisis situation the field boundaries contract and free-energy input/output process is unable to flow. Without the movement of energy, there is nothing to fuel the increasing demands of the forces of labor. Labor may then be experienced as time that is long, "drawn out", and painful, or the experience may be somewhat suspended in time at any one stage. Ms. R's field boundaries are

Diagnosis	Supporting Data	Conflicting Data
	natural desire to move and breathe, and this increases her discomfort.	monitor leads are vital to transmit information about the health and safety of the fetus.
#3	Client does not utilize breathing/relaxation techniques. This increases her discomfort. Ms. R is fighting against the wave of each contraction.	Ms. R is able to experience each contraction and does not manifest uncontrollable behavior. She appears to be coping well.
#4	Client is so focused in on her experience of pain that she is unable to take an active role in her own labor process.	None
#5	Client remains dilated at 5 cm for several hours, even after induction with Pitocin has been started. Does not experience full, strong contractions. She verbalizes that the pain of contraction is centered at the top of the fundus and the pain does not travel down to the pubis.	Contractions are coming at regular intervals and are lasting a normal amount of time.

Nursing Diagnosis	**Rationale**
	constricted: she does not look out of the window or around the room, and she makes no eye contact. She glances at the clock in a worried manner and gazes with a fixed stare at the ceiling during contractions. She remains dilated at 5 cm for several hours, even with Pitocin therapy. Without energy input into the system, she is unable to ''open up'' and allow her labor experience to flow.
6. The client is experiencing decreased field perceptions and altered energy field.	6. Pharmacologically active agents can influence the progression of labor and alter the energy field of the mother and the neonate. Ms. R has received an IM injection of Demerol. The drug works by decreasing perception of pain. In addition, perception of the entire field is depressed. Behavioral manifestations may include dizziness, drowsiness, and euphoria, all psychobiologic states that do not serve to enhance the forces of labor and the birthing process. Nausea and vomiting can be present at delivery, and the infant's physiologic signs may be depressed, with the child requiring oxygen therapy.
7. Energy input into the maternal field is perceived as meaningless information resulting in alteration of space/time orientation.	7. A relationship exists between the rhythmic pattern of the environmental field and that of the human energy field. This interaction affects the client's field and influences the repatterning of her field. Hospital (*i.e.*, environmental) stimuli include the constant beeping tone of the fetal heart monitor, the noises of the buses and traffic going by on Fifth Avenue, and the lowered voices of the doctors, nurses, and other hospital personnel talking about Ms. R, but not to her. Increase in amount, density, and extent of stimuli is also caused by the intermittent presence of a nurse who is cool and distant with the client, two student nurses, and three medical students and their instructor engaged in administering an analgesic epidurally. The unfamiliarity of these sounds, coupled with the number of stimuli present, interact with a maternal field that is experiencing a

Diagnosis	**Supporting Data**	**Conflicting Data**
# 6	Client appears drowsy and less alert after IM injection of Demerol. She is nauseated and has emesis.	None
# 7	Client is withdrawing. Unable to deal with the level of activity in the room. She does not understand why the epidural procedure is taking so long and is so painful.	None

Nursing Diagnosis	**Rationale**
	decreased ability to perceive and organize appropriately, and this results in a state commonly referred to as *sensory overload*.
8. Physiologic systems within maternal field are dysynchronous with structures and functions of the hospital environmental field.	8. The contents of the human energy field are in continuous flux with the contents of the environmental field in a mutual, simultaneous exchange of matter and energy. In the through-put process the changing contents affect the field and the field imposes pattern and organization on the contents. Ms. R was given an enema to empty her bowel of its contents in order to decrease the pressure within the pelvis and the birth canal. In addition, she has been receiving fluids parenterally. These inputs will result in the need for reciprocal energy output (*i.e.*, movement of the bowel and micturition). However, environmental field structures are interacting dysrhythmically with the intake/output of the maternal field and produce disorganizing elements. Owing to the disconcerting presence of the medical team attempting to do the epidural procedure, and the discomfort of the fetal heart monitor, Ms. R is unable to achieve efficient output of her energies. During the increased energy of the transition stage of labor she verbalizes the need to urinate and to defecate, and she is incontinent of urine and feces as she is being transported to the delivery room.

Diagnosis	Supporting Data	Conflicting Data
# 8	Client is unable to void or defecate. She is eventually incontinent of urine and feces.	Client has not requested the bedpan. Her bladder is not distended.

Client-Perceived Areas of Concern (C):

C1.   High degree of pain being caused by forces of labor

C2.   Large amount of time that labor and delivery is making

C3.   Inability to move about freely

C4.   Need for her husband to be beside her

C5.   Need to void and expel enema

Nursing Diagnoses (N):

N1.   Unable to maximize energy of contractions

N2.   Inability to move about decreases maximum wellness

N3.   Constriction of energy field decreases the forces of labor

N4.   Experiencing space/time alteration and consequent sensory overload

N5.   Need to void and expel enema

Combined Client Concerns and Nursing Diagnoses Utilized in Care Plan:

C4

C3, N2

N3

N4

C5, N5

Nursing Care Plan

Diagnosis	Nursing Interventions
C4	Encouraged husband to be part of the birthing process. Allowed him his place beside her, and kept my work to the other side of the bed. I did not ask him to leave the room at any time.
C3,N2	Turned client onto her left side. Raised head of bed when client was lying on her back. I encouraged her to move her legs and to bring her knees up.
N3	Used Therapeutic Touch to encourage intensity and efficiency of client's labor contractions in order to allow labor to progress toward goal of delivery. In addition, I used Therapeutic Touch to calm and relax her emotional state.
N4	Reduced volume of fetal monitor tone. Spoke in normal conversational tones and directly to client. Mentioned what was going on outside the window. Talked about her other children, and drew her husband into conversation. I explained the epidural procedure.
C5,N5	I checked client for distention of bladder.

Rationale

Presence of significant other facilitates client's ability of energy to pass into system. It gave her support and strengthened her emotionally.

Client's remaining immobile for a very long period of time increased discomfort and pain due to poor circulation of blood, oxygen, and nutrients. Sitting upright with knees flexed is a more natural and comfortable position in birthing.

Putting energy into the system enabled the client's labor contractions to flow and allowed for relaxation of constricting boundaries, thereby promoting goal of progression of labor.

Giving concrete meaning to stimuli present in field will decrease meaninglessness of such stimuli. Reducing amount of external stimuli will facilitate inner direction of client's attention on birthing process and will enhance potential for wellness.

Bladder distention causes heightened pressure on the perineum and considerable discomfort.

Evaluation

Client listened to husband's directions *re* breathing, and she relaxed under his guidance.

Client verbalized that she felt more comfortable and could better deal with the contractions when sitting upright.

Labor successful toward goal of delivery.

Conversing with client enabled her to relax and conserve strength between contractions. There was a perceptible decrease in client's anxiety. Client is no longer grimacing or frowning.

Although no distention present, client had not voided nor had she passed the enema. She was not offered the bedpan or checked for voiding often enough, and discomfort and incontinence resulted.

Further Data Needed:

Check for distention and possible impaction of feces during recovery phase.

Discussion of the Case History
Based on Rogers' Conceptual System

Any discussion of the case study that is presented here must proceed on
the prior recognition that the case study is the work of a second-year
college student. This is noted not by way of downgrading the study, for
some of the remarks are full of insight and the analyses are intelligently
handled. Rather, the limitation is that of circumscribed experience. For
instance, the major deficiency of this study as perceived by this writer is
the exclusion of discussion on the principle of resonancy which is
operating actively both during the birthing process and during the
nurse's practice of Therapeutic Touch. However, the explication of this
principle demands a mature and sophisticated grasp of the philosophy
underlying modern science, a knowledge of which the student will
have later in her curriculum.

Throughout the study the orientation is geared toward the
humanistic, rather than the technological, concerns. The plight of Ms. R
is seen as a unified process in which the action results from the human
field of concern and the environmental field in constant flux. Using
this as a frame of reference, the nursing care plan is developed within
the context of the principle of helicy, with recognition given to the
principle of complementarity.

The environmental field (the hospital *in toto*) and the human field
of Ms. R change and are changed by each other. The writer of the case
study, noting the validity of the universe as one of open systems,
develops her nursing therapy on the basis of syntropy, that is, in her
urging of Ms. R to "... ride the wave of contractions" so that the
natural process of labor can be facilitated. She is concerned about the
lack of reciprocity between the human energy field and the
environmental field. The consequent binding of formerly free energy
eventuates in a dysrhythmia which prevents Ms. R from controlling her
own field phenomena, that is, the contractions which are an enactment
of the birthing process itself in reference to the principle of helicy.

This bound energy also distorts the time sense, the energy level is
further depressed, and a state of stasis occurs during which Ms. R's
cervix remains dilated at 5 cm over an extended period. During this
period the human field is deprived of a high-level, mutual,
simultaneous interaction with the environmental field. This dissociation
affects both the human field's response to stimuli, which Ms. R
perceives as meaningless phenomena, and its ability to sensitvely
repattern to meet the changing existential demands made by the
dynamics of the birthing process. The analysis of the situation leads the
writer of the case study to institute Therapeutic Touch as a means of
human field energy interchange. In so using herself therapeutically, the
energy directed toward Ms. R acts synergistically with Ms. R's energy

state. The writer is thus able to help Ms. R to bring her own regenerative abilities into play so that the energy state of the maternal field necessary for the birth of the child is satisfied. The care plan is future-oriented in consonance with the principle of helicy in that suggested considerations are made for the mother's recovery state.

References

1. The Committee on the Function of Nursing: A Program for the Nursing Profession. New York, Macmillan, 1948
2. Rogers ME: Educational Revolution in Nursing. New York, Macmillan, 1961
3. Krieger D: Therapeutic Touch: How to Use Your Hands to Help or to Heal. Englewood Cliffs, Prentice-Hall, 1979
4. Rogers ME: An Introduction to the Theoretical Basis of Nursing, p 44. Philadelphia, FA Davis, 1970
5. Rogers, 1961, *op cit*, pp. 25–27
6. Rogers, 1970, *op cit*, p 47
7. de Broglie L: New Perspectives in Physics, p 68. New York, Basic Books, 1962
8. de Chardin T: The Phenomenon of Man. New York, Harper & Row, 1961
9. Dubos R: Man Adapting. New Haven, Yale University Press, 1965
10. duNoüy L: Human Destiny. New York, Longman's, Green & Co, 1947
11. Herrick CJ: The Evolution of Human Nature. Austin, the University of Texas Press, 1956
12. Miller JG: Living systems: basic concepts. Behavioral Science 10, No. 3:213, 217, 1965
13. Miller JG: Living systems: cross-level hypotheses. Behavioral Science 10, No. 4:407, 1965
14. Mumford L: The Transformation of Man, p 243. New York, Harper & Brothers, 1956
15. Polyani M: Personal Knowledge. Chicago, the University of Chicago Press, 1958
16. Purcell E: Parts and wholes in physics. In Modern Systems Research for the Behavioral Scientist, p 43. Chicago, Aldine Publishing, 1968
17. Rogers, 1970, *op cit*, p 54
18. von Bertalanffy L: The theory of open systems in physics and biology. Science 111:23–25, 1950
19. von Bertalanffy L: General systems theory. Main Currents in Modern Thought 11, No. 4:75–83, 1955
20. Baranski J: Scientific Basis for World Civilization, p 140. Boston, the Christopher Publishing House, 1960
21. duNoüy, 1947, *op cit*, p 90
22. Evans FC: Ecosystems as the basic unit in ecology. In Kormandy EV (ed): Readings in Ecology, p 166. Englewood Cliffs, Prentice-Hall, 1965
23. Hall RD, Fagen RE: Definition of a system. In General Systems Yearbook, 1956
24. Herrick, 1961, *op cit*, p 51

25. Rappaport A: Foreword. In Modern Systems Research for the Behavioral Scientist, p xviii. Chicago, Aldine Publishing, 1968

26. Trincher KS: Biology and Information: Elements of Biological Thermodynamics. Spiegelthal ES (trans). New York, Consultants Bureau Enterprises, 1965

27. von Bertalanffy, 1950, *op cit*, p 25

28. Rogers, 1970, *op cit*, p 59

29. Čapek M: Time in relativity theory: arguments for a philosophy of being. In Fraser JT (ed): The Voices of Time, p 437, 447. New York, George Braziller, 1966

30. deBeauregard OC: Relativity theory: arguments for a philosophy of being. In Fraser JT (ed): Voices of Time, p. 431. New York, George Braziller, 1966

31. de Chardin, 1961, *op cit*, p 49

32. Fischer R (ed): Interdisciplinary Perspectives of Time, p 329. New York, Alfred A Knopf, 1963

33. Fox SW, McCauley RJ: Could life originate now? Natural History, pp 26–30, August-September, 1968

34. Fraser JT (ed): The Voices of Time. New York, George Braziller, 1966

35. Grunbaum A: Philosophical Problems of Space and Time, p 329. New York, Alfred A Knopf, 1963

36. Kalmus H: Organic evolution and time. In Fraser JT (ed): The Voices of Time, p 352. New York, George Braziller, 1966

37. Toulmin S, Goodfield J: The Discovery of Time. New York, Harpers Torchbooks, 1966

38. Rogers, 1970, *op cit*, p 65

39. Ashby WR: Cybernetics, p 54. New York, John Wiley & Sons, 1963

40. von Bertalanffy L: Problems of Life, p. 134. New York, John Wiley & Sons, 1952

41. Cannon WB: The Wisdom of the Body, 2nd ed. New York, Norton Publishing, 1939

42. Dubos, 1965, *op cit*, p 49

43. Herrick, 1956, *op cit*, p 60

44. Frankl VE: Psychotherapy and Existentialism. New York, Simon & Schuster, 1968

45. Maslow AH: Motivation and Personality, p 367. New York, Harper & Row, 1954

46. Polyani, 1958, *op cit*, p 57

47. Sollberger A: Biological Rhythm Research. New York, Elsevier, 1965

48. Whyte LL: The Next Development in Man, p 19. New York, New American Library, 1950

49. Wolf W (ed): Rhythmic functions in the living system. Ann NY Acad Sci V. 98: Art. 4, 1962

50. Rogers, 1970, *op cit*, p 73

51. Clarke AC: The Challenge of the Space Ship, p 145. New York, Ballantine Books, 1961

52. Dement WC: The effect of dream deprivation. Science 131:1705–1707; 132:1420–1422, 1960

53. Frankl V: Man's Search for Meaning. New York, Washington Square Press, 1963

54. Frankl, 1968, *loc cit*
55. Kleitman N: Sleep and Wakefulness, rev ed. Chicago, University of Chicago Press, 1963
56. Langer S: Philosophical Sketches, pp 13, 16. New York, The New American Library of World Literature, 1964
57. Rogers C: Two divergent trends. In May R (ed): Existential Psychology, p 93. New York, Random House, 1961
58. Rogers, 1970, *op cit*, pp 73–77
59. Krieger D: The relationship of touch, with intent to help or to heal, to subjects' in-vivo hemoglobin values: a study in personalized interaction. In Proceedings of the Ninth American Nurses Association Nursing Research Conference. Kansas City, American Nurses Association, 1973
60. Krieger D: Therapeutic touch: the imprimatur of nursing. Am J Nurs 75:784, 1975
61. Krieger, 1975, *op cit*, pp 784–787
62. Peper E, Ancoli S: The two end-points of an EEG continuum of meditation. In Proceedings of the 1977 Biofeedback Research Society of America Conference, Orlando, Florida, 1977
63. Heidt P: An Investigation of the Effects of Therapeutic Touch on Anxiety in Hospitalized Patients. Unpublished doctoral dissertation, New York University, 1979
64. Krieger D: Therapeutic touch: A mode of primary healing based on a holistic concern for man. Journal for Holistic Medicine 1:6–10, 1975
65. Heidt, 1979, *loc cit*
66. Randolph G: The Differences in Physiological Response of Female College Students Exposed to Stressful Stimulus, When Simultaneously Treated by Either Therapeutic Touch or Casual Touch. Unpublished doctoral dissertation, New York University, 1979
67. Rogers, 1970, *op cit*, p 106

9 The Integration of Ancient and Modern Holism: Toward a New Synergy

The Commonalities of Ancient Models of Holism

There is a universal meaning or order in the world of the ancients which is reflected in human beings. When this macrocosmic order is undistorted, the microcosm (man/woman) is in a state of well-being. The potentialities of this order are mobilized through a dual interchange of energies (*yin-yang, ida-pingala,* masculine principle–feminine principle, activity-container or molder of that activity) that affects the individual through a nonmaterial, multidimensional network. This net is vitalized by a universal life energy (*ch'i, prana,* the energy of the *ka*). The life energy is conditioned through the cyclic phenomena of time and becomes apparent as the humors of the body. The combinations of these humors result in the personality characteristics of the individual. Other factors affecting the individual's well-being are climate, seasons of the year, geographical location, the individual's nutritional status, age, sex, and temperament, and the manner in which he or she conducts the daily acts of living. The life process was thought to be on a continuum that transcended death.

A Consensus of Modern Models of Holism

Within the contemporary holistic health frame of reference, there is general agreement that the universe is syntropic (*i.e.,* a net of open systems tending toward order). Through philosophical deduction,[1] scientific systems analysis,[2] and quantum analysis,[3] as well as through personal accounts of transpersonal experience,[4] it is acknowledged that there is a universe of meaning, a state of consciousness that transcends the usual abilities of human perception. When a person enters this transcendent state in full consciousness, there is a heightened sense of well-being and an intimate knowledge of the basic oneness of the universe.[5] When, however, a person enters the transcendent state before being personally and fully prepared, or enters this state of consciousness by chance, life-threatening illness may follow.[6]

There is also agreement that the basic substances of all physical being, force, and matter are but different transformations of the same phenomena, reality being momentarily caught in the web of relationships of dynamic and patterned processes. These interactional latticeworks are relativistic in nature and are space–time-oriented within a multidimensional matrix in constant flux.

Light (through photon conversion during the process of photosynthesis) is considered to be the basis of life-giving energy. For this reason, the electromagnetic field, the basic unit of which is the photon and the field of which is coextensive with the universe, is thought to be fundamentally involved in the life process.[7]

Human behavior has been demonstrated to be significantly influenced by pulses of rhythmic energies the sources of which are either in the environment (exogenous rhythms, such as those that underlie day–night alteration, seasonal changes, *etc.*) or within the individual (endogenous rhythms). They are known to affect particularly chemical fluids and hormones in the body structure and reactions between deep brain structures and the cortex.[8]

The study of the ingestion of essential food components as a means of sustaining the well-being of life through a competent knowledge of nutrition coupled with a conscious philosophy of self-regulation is still in the gestational stages,[9,10] and death has only recently been widely recognized to be intrinsic to the continuum of life.[11-13] However, the effects of climate, geographical location,[14,15] and environment[16,17] are receiving increasing attention and understanding.

In brief, these bits of information form the major facets of the theoretical background against which the rationale of the current holistic health movement is graphically portrayed. Although arrived at by other, empirical, means, they serve at least two purposes. In a general way they substantiate the bases of ancient models of holism to a considerable degree, and they translate these concepts into the modern idiom.

Principles of Holistic Health Practice

Responsibility for Self

A major key to the principles that underlie holistic health practice is the recognition that the physical, psychomental, spiritual, and interactive condition of a person is that individual's personal responsibility because it is the individual alone who makes the decision of how to react under stress.[18] When the pattern of decision leads to disorders over time, it becomes part of the function of the holistic health practioner to analyze the dysfunctional pattern of behavior and to assist the person to repattern his or her responses in a more life-affirmative manner.

"Listen" for Body Cues

A holistic health practice that appears to have increasing validity is to teach the individual to become aware of stressors by learning to "listen" to his or her body for selective cues when the person is stressed (*i.e.,* to recognize how the body–mind reacts under stress).[19] Once these body–mind cues are brought to conscious awareness, or are anchored, they are dealt with in a decisive and constructive manner by the individual learning to reframe his or her physiologic and psychologic response pattern.[20]

Change in Self-Concept
Facilitates a Change in Life-Style

When an individual finds that he or she need not be a passive pawn in his or her own health care but can actively and responsibly participate in the process of self-healing, a discriminative change in self-concept can occur. This altered concept of self often facilitates a fundamental change in the individual's belief system. The knowledgeable holistic health practitioner will take advantage of this decisive change in perspective to encourage the person to carefully examine his or her life-style and to institute any necessary corrective changes or practices in the direction of an actualization of personal potential for high-level wellness. A sound basis for this examination is a life history review, such as Travis' *Wellness Inventory,*[21] which can be restructured to meet the requirements of nursing diagnosis and a subsequent nursing care plan of holistic health practices. In developing this plan it is important to consider the timing of the life-style changes that are introduced to the person. These life-style changes should be paced so that the experiences the person undergoes, as well as the world view to which he or she is exposed, are constructively integrated within the unique framework of that individual so as to enhance his or her life.

Responding to the Paradigm Shift

The success of a holistic health orientation in the individual rests upon the individual's ungrudging ability to deeply examine previous assumptions, values, goals, and relationships, and to radically change his or her world view. In one of the most perceptive and thorough analyses of the contemporary holistic movement as a new cultural awakening, Ferguson recently reported on questionnaire returns of a sample of 189 persons engaged in current social transformations.[22] She was able to differentiate four stages which occurred as these people went through the transformative process inherent in the enactment of a holistic world view in their lives:

1. The initial point of entry for the individual can occur anywhere in the holistic health practice spectrum: meditation, autogenic training, biofeedback, or whatever. Its characteristic mark, however, is that whatever a person chooses serves to jolt that person's previous conception of "how things are," of the reality that gives meaning to that person's world. In their initial enthusiasm, persons at this stage may ardently believe that only the practice in which they are personally involved is the answer to the problems of the world. However, continued involvement in that particular method may be only partially fulfilling or the person may realize that the method may not hold the same interest for everyone.

2. This leads the person to explore other practices, to do what Ferguson calls "comparison shopping." During this period of exploration, the person tests the measure of various practices against his or her individual needs and expectations. Should there be a close fit, an in-depth study may occur.

3. As the seeker's interest deepens, he or she begins to integrate the newly acquired knowledge into his or her life-style. Ferguson notes that this period of integration is also a period of crucial personal decisions because the individual realizes that he or she has changed and that in order to be viable a new world view must be reflected in his or her life-style. This implementation of a decision to change may be steeped in feelings of inadequacy, fear of loss of familiar relationships and habits, and timidity in structuring new values and goals. This may also be a more reflective period and, if the person persists, may eventuate in in-depth studies, particularly about subjects concerned with shifts in states of consciousness.

4. Finally, in this pursuit of self-knowledge, the person begins to gain personal knowledge about the power within the self and intimations of how this power may be used for self and for others. Personal insights (that it is when conflict, pain, tension, and fear are confronted that the transformation process may begin) may illuminate his or her studies. In time the person may come to realize that one can pass on this knowledge to others who are also seeking. If this knowledge is passed on, that person then becomes

part of a network of information, one of the group involved in what Ferguson calls the "Aquarian Conspiracy," a conspiracy that makes transformation possible for those who are avidly seeking a creative alternative to the old social forms. Ferguson calls the emergence of these networks ". . . a new social form . . . an unprecedented source of power for individuals."[23] This can be so, for it is the wise one that knows, and knows that he or she knows, and it is the compassionate one who will freely share that knowledge.

The Renaissance Nurse

It has been the underlying purpose of Part 2 of this book to show that the farther reaches of holistic health nursing practices hold personal implications the eddies of which may be as far-reaching as their depths are profound. The singular nature of these implications for the individual nurse involved in these holistic health practices must at least be acknowledged; however, mere acknowledgment in itself will never get one to those farther reaches. To be involved, to really understand, one must have personal knowledge, for the crux of the holistic experience lies in its transformative elements.

Sometimes a catch-phrase aids in the realization of what is needed for the facilitation of this particular change, and so, for the purposes of this summation of Part 2, I would like to offer for consideration a term I coined in 1972 which has been used since then by many nurses. At that time, at the close of the revolutions of the 1960s, it became evident that the nurse of the future would face a radically different world than had previous nurses. As a professional person, there was only one way the nurse could intervene in another's health care, and that was from a knowledgeable stance. With the continuing implosion of information from all fields of human inquiry still to crest, it was nevertheless becoming apparent that our picture of reality was not in phase with reality as science was now perceiving it. Nurses in particular needed to apply themselves diligently to the understanding of the key elements of this new knowledge if they were to comprehend human beings accurately within the perspective of the rapidly advancing frontiers of knowledge. Admittedly, because of the complexity of the human condition, the task would be of heroic proportions.

The measure of the nurse who would be able to assimilate these broad principles as they emerged from the growing edge of information would be characterized by the ability to facilely use "whole-brain" thinking. That is, the nurse would be as equally able to appreciate the aesthetic qualities of humans as to analyze their being. Moreover, this person would be able to synthesize his or her conclusions and to articulate them in a holistic nursing care plan, research proposal, or teaching outline.

The Renaissance of the fifteenth and sixteenth centuries was a pivotal age, as is the present. It was an age that celebrated the dignity of man, an age in which there was an explosion of creative energy, an age that revolutionized learning. What was necessary at the present time, I thought, was a need for understanding such as that which urged the people of the Renaissance to make themselves knowledgeable about all appropriate and significant facets of their world. I named such a nurse the *Renaissance Nurse*, taking the initials *R.N.* from the traditional title, registered nurse. The Renaissance was a time that marked the decline of holism as a living philosophy (see Chap. 5). It would be very appropriate that the R.N. of a new age, the Renaissance Nurse, revitalize the philosophy of holism through the humanism of nursing.

It is the Renaissance Nurse who is at the forefront of the holistic health nursing movement. The Renaissance Nurse humanizes and individualizes nursing practice. His or her understanding of holism provides a context for nursing therapy and nursing prognosis so that a nursing care plan (really a "nurse-caring plan") is an enactment of process based on the flow of the individual client's healing of self.

The Renaissance Nurse teaches the client appropriate techniques for centering, meditation, relaxation, or imagery—all of which can be done while the client is in bed, if necessary—and punctuates the client's rehabilitation with shared teaching–learning experiences on body awareness, yoga, neuro-linguistics, or biofeedback. One of the most innovative uses of the latter by nurses dealing with people in deep psychologic crisis, for instance, has been the adaptation of biofeedback techniques to facial muscles to help persons who have suffered profound emotional trauma. These persons have so dissociated themselves from the traumatic experiences that they can no longer cry. In teaching these clients biofeedback techniques that will stimulate the mobilization of the facial muscles involved in crying, there has been a significantly high success rate of these people being able once again to engage spontaneously in the natural act of crying.

The Renaissance Nurse strives to synthesize information about the client so that there can be a fuller appreciation of the depth of the problems in the situation as well as a reality-oriented perspective on their relative importance. High ability in pattern recognition is another mark of the Renaissance Nurse because it is the configuration of the clues about the client's health (rather than the individual bits of information such as laboratory reports, intake–output records, *etc.*) that give the best indications of the client's state of health and potential for change.

The clients of the Renaissance Nurse learn that illness can be an opportunity for the discovery of meaning in their lives, and they are encouraged to be active and innovative in their own self-healing. Their quest for high-level wellness becomes a joint activity with the Renaissance Nurse in which they are urged toward individual, knowledgeable responsibility for self.

In life-style and world view, the Renaissance Nurse is future-oriented, committed to personal participation, open to creative change, appreciative of order and meaning in the universe, and accepting of the responsibility to foster balance in the health orientation of those for whom he or she has a nurse-caring plan.

References

1. Merrill-Wolff F: The Philosophy of Consciousness Without an Object: Reflections of the Nature of Transcendental Consciousness, pp 93–265. New York, Julian Press, 1973
2. Tart CT: States of Consciousness, pp 272–286. New York, EP Dutton, 1975
3. Capra F: The Tao of Physics, pp 130 –143. Berkeley, Shambhala, 1975
4. Yü LK: The Secrets of Chinese Meditation, 2nd ed, pp 191–218. New York, Samuel Weiser, 1971
5. Yü, 1971, *loc cit*
6. Krishna G: Kundalini: the Evolutionary Energy in Man. Berkeley, Shambhala, 1971
7. Krasnovsky AA: The evolution of photochemical electron transfer systems. In Kimball AP, Oro J (eds): Prebiotic and Biochemical Evolution, pp 209–211. New York, American Elsevier, 1971
8. Sollberger A: Biological Rhythms Research, pp 310 –314. New York, American Elsevier, 1965
9. Ballentine R: Diet and Nutrition: a Holistic Approach, pp 480–588. Honesdale, Himalayan International Institute, 1978
10. Mackarness R: Eating Dangerously: the Hazards of Hidden Allergies. New York, Harcourt, Brace & Jovanovich, 1976
11. Kübler-Ross E: Death: the Final Stage of Growth. Englewood Cliffs, Prentice-Hall, 1975
12. Moody RA: Life After Life. Covington, Mockingbird Press, 1975
13. Osis K, Haraldsson E: At the Hour of Death. New York, Avon Books, 1977
14. Krieger AP, Reed EJ: Biological impact of small air ions. Science 193:1209–1213, 1976
15. Soyka F: The Ion Effect. New York, EP Dutton, 1977
16. Ott JN: Responses of psychological and physiological functions to environmental radiation stress. Journal of Learning Disabilities, June, 1968
17. Hammond EC, Selikoff IJ (eds): Public control of environmental health hazards. Ann NY Acad Sci Vol 329 (entire volume), 1979
18. Pelletier KR: Mind as Healer, Mind as Slayer, p 16. New York, Delacorte Press, 1976
19. Bandler R, Grindler J: Frogs Into Princes: Neuro-Linguistic Programming. Real People Press, Box F, Moab, Utah 84532, 1979

20. Pelletier, 1977, *op cit*, pp 33–35
21. Travis J: Wellness Inventory. Wellness Center, Mill Valley, CA, 1975
22. Ferguson M: The Aquarian Conspiracy: Personal and Social Transformation in the 1980's, pp 60–63. Los Angeles, JP Tarcher, 1980
23. Ferguson, 1980, *op cit*, p 17

Part 3
Clinical Papers of the Holistic Health Perspective

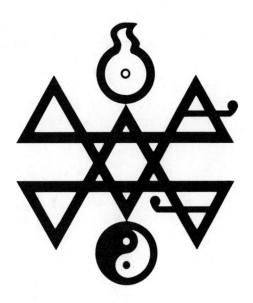

10 The Creative Nurse: A Holistic Perspective

Dolores Krieger

As a society, we are only now emerging from the shock suffered by both young and old following the revolutions of the 1960s, and from the sense of personal powerlessness that was characteristic of the early 1970s. A new message is coming forth, however, which states that we can help each other, we can help ourselves. A new age of understanding is dawning that has the philosophy of holism as its context, an age in which human beings can intelligently cooperate with nature and with each other.

The method for achieving this state of being is not to submerge one's self in the collectivity, the mass, but rather the method is one of unique and personal effort toward the conscious realization and actualization of one's own potential.[1,2] This individuation process comes to fruition in the seeking of self-knowledge, and in the seeking comes the recognition of the unitive base of one's own nature, a unitive network that uniquely structures the perspective of its numberless connectivities to both other human beings and to the universe. It is in this holistic view that the power of the orientation of the new age lies. It is through the integration and complementarity of consciousness and the unconscious that occurs as a result of the individuation process that the most creative state of the individual psyche is fostered.[3]

Creative, holistic nursing practice offers an opportunity for this kind of intelligent cooperation in the interest of human beings, a need I have come to call the *need-to-help*. It is theorized that the need-to-help wells up from the same psychodynamic depths from which arose the stimuli that guided early men and women not merely to mate, but to form the nuclear family in which the attributes of love and caring and protection from harm are nurtured. It is probably the most humane of human characteristics, and lies very close to the central incentives that motivate people to become nurses.

In the nursing act, this need-to-help expresses itself in many ways. In its most constructive out-working, the deeply human qualities of empathy, compassion, and a desire to lift a little the veil of pain and suffering that seems to clothe the human condition find expression.

These altruistic characteristics, frequently spoken of as *caritas* and *agape*, help provide dosages of what Pitrim A. Sorokin has called "the vitamin of love" to persons who are ill and in need. This act of transpersonal love has been a hallmark of nursing, a tradition that goes back to the medieval days of the hospice.

Therapeutic Touch

One of the uniquely human acts that permeates almost every phase of nursing is characterized by the touching of another in an act that incorporates an intent to help or to heal the person so touched. Over the past ten years, I have been engaged in nursing research in a form of touch that I have come to call *Therapeutic Touch*.

What It Is

Therapeutic Touch derives from, but is not the same as, the ancient art of the laying-on of hands. The major points of difference between Therapeutic Touch and the laying-on of hands are methodological: Therapeutic Touch has no religious base as does the laying-on of hands; it is a conscious, intentional act; it is based on research findings; and Therapeutic Touch does not require a declaration of faith from the healee (patient) for it to be effective.

The methods used in the act of Therapeutic Touch appear to the casual observer to be quite simple. However, much as other complex human acts, such as seeing, are at first thought to be simple, upon serious study, these methods are found to be exceedingly complex. There are many levels of expertise in the practice of Therapeutic Touch, but basically Therapeutic Touch is an act which nurses engage in quite naturally in the course of their nursing practice. On the whole, our society supports a no-touch culture. But nurses are a notable exception to these taboos. We are allowed to touch, we are allowed intimacies no other profession is allowed. It could be said that touch is almost a badge of the nursing profession; it is its imprimatur, so to speak. Therefore, I, as a nurse, have found this therapeutic use of touch to be a very meaningful experience, a creative avenue for the expression of my own nursing expertise, and a challenging arena in which to test my conceptions about the focus of nursing: human beings.

My studies really began as a student nurse when I was learning to accept beliefs that the restorative processes in humans were limited. Most readers, I am sure, have known the sense of dissatisfaction that surrounds this belief, and several of us would be willing to admit to instances in which we have secretly questioned a situation in which it had been decreed that "nothing more can be done." I was very lucky to have had an opportunity to examine these questions closely.

Some years ago, it was my good fortune to be asked by a friend to assist in a clinic conducted by a very well-known healer, Oskar Estebany,[4] on one of his annual visits to this country. My job was to help with the case histories, to take various vital signs on the patients, and to help to collate material at the end of the study. People with a wide variety of diseases, many of which were in advanced stages, came to these clinics from all over the country. I had many excellent opportunities to observe the interaction of these healees (patients) with the healer quite closely and under a variety of circumstances. What I saw was not startling. The atmosphere in the room in which the healing took place was friendly and quiet. Conversation, when it occurred, was natural and spontaneous. Estebany's touch was light and relaxed, with no unusual passes or maneuvers. To a casual observer, it may have seemed as though nothing was happening, but with time a significant number of these healees got better. Most of them had verified medical histories of illness and had been referred by medical doctors who, in turn, verified their patients' improved conditions when they returned to them for check-ups. Nothing in either my previous education or in my experience had prepared me for these kinds of findings; and so, remembering my own questionings, I decided to study this phenomenon in considerable depth.

Early Studies by Biochemists

A thorough search of the literature from various Western countries revealed little in the way of substantive studies, and of these studies only two, both by biochemists, had been dealt with as rigorously as demanded by scientific methodologies.

One of the biochemists, Grad, of McGill University, had studied the effects of healing by the laying-on of hands on plants.[5] In Grad's studies, barley seeds, which sprout rapidly, were soaked in saline solution before the experiment to simulate a "sick" condition in the seeds. Interestingly, the seeds themselves were not directly treated, for Grad set the study up so that the water that would irrigate the samples of seeds would be the medium that would carry the effect of the healing, if indeed there was such an effect. To do this, Grad set up three situations. In the first case, he had the same healer I mentioned above, Estebany, hold flasks of water and do to the flasks whatever it was that he did when treating a person with the laying-on of hands. Then this water was used to irrigate the first sample of barley seeds. In the second case, a group of disinterested medical students went through the same maneuvers as Estebany, but with other flasks of water, and they did not do laying-on of hands. Then this water was used to irrigate a second sample of barley seeds. In the third case, plain untreated water was used to irrigate a third sample of barley seeds. Grad reported that the seeds watered from flasks held by Estebany sprouted earlier and the plants grew taller and had a greater amount of chlorophyll in them. These findings were such that they could have happened by chance less than once in a thousand times.

Grad's study was done in the early 1960s. In the late 1960s, another biochemist, Dr. M. Justa Smith, then of Rosary Hill College, was intrigued and stimulated by Grad's studies, and she decided to develop further research on the laying-on of hands. Her assumption was that if an energy change occurred during healing by any means whatsoever, that change should be apparent at the enzymatic level of the organism, for it is the enzymes that are crucial to the basic metabolism of the body. Estebany cooperated with Dr. Smith in a double-blind study using the enzyme trypsin as the test object to see whether indeed treatment by the laying-on of hands would have a significant effect on enzymes.[6]

In the study, Dr. Smith set up four conditions. One fraction of the trypsin solution was subjected to high ultra-violet rays to simulate a "sick" condition. This sample as well as an unaltered sample (*i.e.*, "healthy") were held in test tubes by Estabany for 75 minutes each day. A third fraction was subjected to an exceedingly high magnetic field (13,000 gauss), and a fourth fraction was held as a control without being given any treatment. In solution, enzymes decompose quickly. For this reason, the research design called for many daily runs, with fresh samples of enzyme solution being used each day. The research findings showed that for the first hour of the daily runs there were high correlations between the relative percent of activity in the samples held by Estebany and those subjected to the high magnetic field. However, after the first hour, the enzymes held by Estebany significantly exceeded the sample exposed to the high magnetic field.

Study With Hemoglobin as Variable

While analyzing these studies for clues for further research, I recalled literature I had read several years earlier while I was doing studies on comparative religion, and I thought it might have relevance for my quest. This literature was derived from the East, particularly from India[7] and Tibet.[8] Briefly, it states that life energies in humans, which we in the West call *animation* or *vigor*, are an expression of an energy system called *prana*, which is said to be solar in origin and to be intimately connected to oxygen. The literature states that healthy people have an overabundance of *prana*, whereas sick people have a deficit, and it also notes that *prana* uses the breathing, the blood, or the nerves as conductors.

In my study of healers who used the laying-on of hands, I was very impressed by the concentrated sense of intentionality that suffused the healer even though neither physical strain nor stress was apparent. It therefore appeared plausible that this personalized interaction was a consciously motivated act. I felt that some considerable support for this assumption of intentionality was to be found in the literature of hatha yoga and tantric yoga, which states that pranic flow is amenable to direction and manipulation by what we in the West would call "mind control."[9]

Therefore, the conceptualization that was fundamental to this study was founded on the assumption of the human as an open system. It conceived the healer as being an individual whose health gave him or her access to an overabundance of *prana*. The strong sense of commitment and intentionality to help ill people gave this person a certain control over the projection of this vital energy. The act of healing then would entail the channeling of this energy flow by the healer for the well-being of the ill person.

Integrating this literature from the East with the studies noted above, I selected hemoglobin, a blood component, as the dependent variable in a study of the laying-on of hands. I chose hemoglobin because it is one of the body's most sensitive indicators of oxygen uptake and also because it is quite accessible for study of bioenergetic changes that might underlie this mode of healing. As noted above, Eastern literature suggests that *prana* is intrinsic in what we in the West call the *oxygen molecule*. Another reason for the choice of hemoglobin concerned one of the findings in Grad's study on barley seeds which demonstrated an increase in the chlorophyll content of the sprouts that had been irrigated with water treated by the healer. It happens that the biochemical configuration of the porphyrin structure of hemoglobin, a structure that is crucial to hemoglobin's function as a highly efficient conveyor of oxygen to the tissues, resembles its homologue in chlorophyll on several counts. Because there is this close similarity between hemoglobin and chlorophyll, it seemed reasonable that hemoglobin would be an appropriate test object in human subjects. In addition, Dr. Smith's study indicated that enzyme systems were sensitive to the laying-on of hands. Because there are several enzyme systems crucial to both the biosynthesis and the functioning of hemoglobin, it was felt that hemoglobin would be a sensitive indicator of the energy change that Dr. Smith established as requisite for healing to take place.

Using hemoglobin values as the dependent variable, I drew up the following research design. I designated a group of sick people as an experimental group; the members of this sample would be treated by a healer using the laying-on of hands. It was my good fortune to have Mr. Estebany serve as the healer in the first three of these studies. A second, comparable group had no such treatment and served as the control group. Pretest samples of blood were then taken from both groups to determine whether the hemoglobin values of both groups were equivalent, and upon analysis it was determined that there was no significant difference between the means of these groups. I also controlled for other possible intervening variables, such as age, sex, diet, medications, recent trauma, habitual smoking, and some biorhythms. My hypothesis was that there would be a significant change in the hemoglobin values of the experimental group following treatment by the healer, whereas there would be no significant change in the hemoglobin values of the control group after a comparable period of time. With the exception of treatment of the members of the experimental group by the laying-on of hands, other conditions for both groups were the same.

In 1971, I conducted a pilot study that indicated the feasability of a full-scale study. In 1972, I conducted a full-scale study in which there were 43 persons in the experimental group and 33 persons in the control group. The hypotheses were upheld by a confidence level exceeding .01; that is, there was less than one possibility in a hundred that the research findings could have happened by chance. I reported my findings to my own professional group, at the American Nurses Association Ninth Conference of the Council of Nurse Researchers, and later at research conferences of other professions.

Profiting by the critiques, both within nursing and from other disciplines, I repeated my study in 1973. The Wallace study on the physiologic effects of transcendental mediation had been reported in the interim.[10] Therefore, in order to check whether unbeknownst to me there had inadvertently been intervention either by the practice of meditation by my sample subjects or through the kind of ventilatory exercises that are taught to persons who undergo chest surgery or the kind of breathing exercises done in yoga, I controlled for both meditation and ventilatory exercises in this replicatory study in addition to the variables that had been controlled for in the previous studies. For this study there were 46 persons in the experimental group and 29 persons in the control group. My hypotheses were again upheld, this time by a probability that indicated that the research findings could have happened by chance less than once in a thousand times.

Healing by Laying-on of Hands

During the course of these studies I grew curious about the process of healing by the laying-on of hands and learned how to do it under the tutelage of Dora Van Gelder Kunz.[11] In time I found that I could elicit reactions in healees similar to those stated in the literature. Specifically, the healees would feel heat in the tissues underlying the area over which I held my hands; they would feel profoundly relaxed; and they reported a sense of well-being.

The conceptualization that I now began to develop from experiencing all of the above ran something like this: I realized that my basic assumption was that human beings are open systems, that they appear to be a nexus of all fields of which life partakes; that is, human beings are the nexus of the inorganic fields as well as the organic fields, the psychic as well as the conceptual fields (the electrodynamic being only one interface of the whole), and as such they are exquisitely sensitive to wave phenomena (*i.e.,* energy). I saw the healer to be an individual whose personal health gave him or her access to an overabundance of *prana* (the healer's health being an indication that he or she was in highly efficient interaction with the significant field forces) and whose motivation and intentionality gave him or her a certain control over the projection of *prana* for the well-being of other.

On the physical level I deduced that this projection occurs by electron-transfer resonance. The resonance would act in the service of the ill person to reestablish the vital flow in this open system—to restore, as it were, unimpeded communication of the individual's field complex with that of the environment. Given this, as all literature on healing agrees, the healees can really heal themselves.

Further theoretical analysis of this model suggested the hypothesis that if the healee was able to sustain this threshold (*i.e.,* if his or her own recuperative powers were activated), he or she could achieve full recovery. However, if the integrity of the system was too fragmented to fully respond once it was on its own, that person's recovery would be relatively less, or after an initial spurt he or she might relapse, or there might not be any apparent effect.

I found that frequently when I treated a healee his or her healing processes were measurably accelerated, and when I took blood samples from the healee it would be found that the hemoglobin values had significantly changed. It occurred to me that since I could do this, then perhaps this type of healing is not something only a few chosen people could do. Perhaps this type of healing was a natural potential in human beings that could be actualized under the conditions mentioned above; that is, the person had the intent to help or to heal, he was constructively motivated in his intention, and he was able to confront himself, by which I mean that he was able to answer to himself the question "Why do I want to play the role of healer?"

Study Conducted in 1974

I decided to test out this notion, and in 1974 I repeated the entire study in which Kunz, whose help to me is noted above, and I taught registered nurses a variant of the laying-on of hands for which I have coined the term *Therapeutic Touch*. In its final form, there were 32 registered nurses in this study and 64 patients. The study was done in hospitals and other health facilities in metropolitan New York. The design was such that there were 16 nurses in the experimental group and 16 nurses in the control group, and each nurse had 2 patients. In the experimental group, the nurses treated their patients with Therapeutic Touch, whereas the nurses in the control group did only routine nursing practices on their patients. The patients in both groups were matched; that is, there were similar characteristics in both groups on all of the major variables noted above. In addition, because of the structured nature of hospitals and health facilities, I was able to add the following delimitations:

1. I requested that each of the participating nurses, whether in the experimental group or in the control group, abide by the Patient's Bill of Rights; that is, that they obtain individual informed consent from their patients for their participation in a research study, although of course the patients themselves did not know to which group they would be randomly assigned.

2. Each nurse was assured of the cooperation as well as the consent of their patients' attending physicians (for instance, the blood samples had to be obtained through medical order).

3. The consent and cooperation of the facility's department of nursing was also obtained.

4. Where there was a board of research review in the facility, I asked that a formal request for approval of the use of the facilities be instituted, and appropriate materials were made available for presentation.

5. To reduce possible bias, I further stipulated that the laboratory technicians at the health facilities not be told that a study was in progress.

6. In the study I only included data for which the same type of blood analysis equipment was used (Coulter).

The hypotheses were essentially similar to those stated in the previous studies; specifically, that the hemoglobin values and the hematocrit ratios of the patients in the experimental group (who would be treated with Therapeutic Touch) would significantly change from their pretreatment values. However, the blood values of the control group (who would be treated with routine nursing care only) would demonstrate no essential difference over a comparable period of time and under comparable conditions. This proved to be the case, the level of confidence being such that the research findings could have happened by chance less than once in a thousand times ($p < .001$).[12]

Results of Therapeutic Touch Studies

One of the valuable spin-offs of subjecting Therapeutic Touch to the rigors of Western research methodologies on the one hand and to the formality of developing its theoretical content within the traditional structuring of an academic environment on the other has been the emergence of the inherent strength of this therapeutic use of touch (which has a written history of over 5,000 years and a pictorial history in cave paintings going back 15,000 years) that is essentially human in nature. I have often thought that it is perhaps one of the most humane of human therapeutics. Another asset of subjecting Therapeutic Touch to these stringent controls has been that Therapeutic Touch has been exposed to constant objective observation and further study by both this writer and, more importantly, my colleagues in nursing and in other professions, as well as by both master's degree candidates and doctoral students. There have been both replications of the original research and extensions of that research that are currently in progress. Close scrutiny of the physiologic effects of patients being treated by Therapeutic Touch have elicited four reliable observable physical changes that occur in these healees. These changes essentially constitute a relaxation response and occur as follows: (1) the first observable change noted is that the voice level of the healee drops several decibels; (2) there is then a noted change in respirations in which the respirations become slower and deeper; (3) following this, an audible sign of relaxation occurs and is most usually signaled by a deep inhalation, a sigh, or an actual statement such as "I feel so relaxed"; (4) another interesting sign is that a peripheral flush will be noted in the healee; this is a generalized slight pinking-up of the skin that occurs throughout the body but is most readily perceived on the healee's face. The question of why this apparent dilation of the peripheral vascular system occurs has not as yet been studied, but that it does indeed happen seems irrefutable at this time.[13] This above-noted relaxation response holds considerable promise for further study and is most certainly a major reason why stress-related disorders respond very well to Therapeutic Touch, as does pain, and possibly may form the basis for the accelerated healing that can take place through Therapeutic Touch. At this time, the delimitations of Therapeutic Touch are not fully known. This, of course, is a function of the many unknowns at this time of both Therapeutic Touch and of the full stature of human beings themselves.

Since this study was completed, I have proposed and have had accepted a graduate course at the master's degree level at New York University which has been designed to formally teach the therapeutic use of human field interaction and to develop theory concerned with its underlying bioenergetics and psychodynamics. The course is currently finishing its sixth year, and I teach it in both the Fall and the Spring semesters. The course is academically structured with appropriate objectives, catalogue description, course outline, prerequisites, grade requirements, bibliographies, and so on. Although it was the first such course within an accredited master's degree curriculum in the United States , several of its graduates are now setting up courses of their own, and so the principles and concepts of Therapeutic Touch are permeating the health field. Currently there is a survey in progress to determine how many universities in the United States and Canada are using Therapeutic Touch in their curricula. The last survey, in Spring 1979, found that there were 33 universities using Therapeutic Touch at that time. In addition, Therapeutic Touch is taught in innumerable professional continuing education courses at universities and in in-service programs at hospitals and other health facilities. In these latter settings, nurses use Therapeutic Touch throughout the whole spectrum of their holistic nursing practices as a natural extension of their professional skills.

As has been noted briefly in Chapter 8, there have been several studies on Therapeutic Touch which have been completed by the time of this writing. These studies have demonstrated that besides the change in hemoglobin values and hematocrit ratios noted above, treatment by Therapeutic Touch significantly affects brain waves[14] and state–anxiety,[15] and brings about a generalized relaxation response.[16] At this writing, replications are in process both in this country and abroad. At least four studies currently under way indicate the innovative ways in which Therapeutic Touch may be used. These researchers are studying the relationship between treatment in brain-injured patients and their consequent intracranial pressure, qualitative changes that occur in the consciousness of practitioners of Therapeutic Touch, attitudinal changes subsequent to treatment by Therapeutic Touch of parents of abused children, and changes in family-centered relationships that occur when, during childbirth using the Lamaze method, the father of the child plays the role of healer and does Therapeutic Touch to the mother. The last is a two-part study in which physiologic changes in the mother and child are also being studied. As noted previously, at the time of this writing two doctoral dissertations on Therapeutic Touch have been completed for the Ph.D. degree in nursing research and theoretical development,[17,18] and several others are in progress in nursing and in other fields.

Because the conceptual basis of helping or healing by Therapeutic Touch includes the assumption that the person playing the role of healer acts as a human support system, there is also a tacit acknowledgment that the individual so engaged has license for individual interpretation. This allows for a wide margin of unique and creative involvement by the healer in this highly personalized therapeutic interaction and carries with it, of course, recognition of the concomitant responsibility for such innovative practice.

However, as noted above, the fully creative person is the person who is truly whole, who has accepted not only the obvious, outer trappings of his or her involvement in the human condition, but also the cognizance of the dynamics that relate that person meaningfully to the continuum of his or her own innermost being as well as to the intrinsic connectivities which bind him or her to the universe and *vice versa*. As one internalizes this total, holistic orientation, the sphere of personal accountability quite naturally transforms itself to accommodate that larger, more human perspective.

References

1. Singer J: Boundaries of the Soul, pp 157–159. Garden City, Doubleday, 1973
2. Maslow A: The Farther Reaches of Human Nature, pp 25–41. New York, Viking Press, 1972
3. Progoff I: Jung, Synchronicity and Human Destiny, pp 90–91. New York, Julian Press, 1973
4. Sullivan GB: Oskar's exotic hands. Saturday Review, pp 17–18. March, 1973
5. Grad B: A telekinetic effect on plant growth. II: Experiments involving treatment of saline in stoppered bottles. International Journal of Parapsychology 6:473–498, 1964
6. Smith MJ: Paranormal effects on enzyme activity. Human Dimensions 1:15–19, 1972
7. Thakkur CG: Introduction to Ayurveda. New York, Asi Publishers, 1974
8. Kunzang RRJ (trans): Tibetan Medicine. Berkeley, University of California Press, 1973
9. Eliade M: Yoga: Immortality and Freedom, pp 151–152. Princeton, Princeton University Press, 1969
10. Wallace RK: Physiological effects of Transcendental Meditation. Science 167:1751–1754, 1971
11. Karagulla S: Breakthrough to Creativity, pp 123–146. Los Angeles, DeVoss, 1967
12. Krieger D: Therapeutic Touch: the imprimatur of nursing. Am J Nurs 75:784–787, 1975
13. Krieger D: Therapeutic Touch: How to Use Your Hands to Help or to Heal, pp 75–76. Englewood Cliffs, Prentice-Hall, 1979
14. Peper E, Ancoli S: The two end-points of an EEG continuum of meditation. Proceedings of the 1977 Biofeedback Research Society of America Conference, Orlando, Florida, 1977
15. Heidt P: An Investigation of the Effects of Therapeutic Touch on Anxiety in Hospitalized Patients. Unpublished doctoral dissertation, New York University, 1979

16. Krieger D: Therapeutic Touch: a mode of primary healing based on a holistic concern for man. Journal for Holistic Medicine 1:6–10, 1975
17. Heidt, 1979, *loc cit*
18. Randolph G: The Differences in Physiological Response of Female College Students Exposed to Stressful Stimulus, When Simultaneously Treated by Either Therapeutic Touch or Casual Touch. Unpublished doctoral dissertation, New York University, 1979

11 Listening: An Essay on the Nature of Holistic Assessment

Janet A. Macrae

Within the holistic framework, a human being is a multidimensional being—a complex, dynamic web of interrelated aspects. Each person is a pattern, so to speak, within the larger fabric of the universe—one melody within a universal symphony.

Just as the universe as a whole operates under natural laws, so does humanity. Within the dynamic pattern of humanness, there is a strong tendency toward order, health, and fulfillment. Dr. Ira Progoff describes this inner drive as the "directive principle" inherent within each individual.[1] He writes that this principle is observable throughout the natural world, as all living beings seem to be drawn in a direction that fulfills the potentialities of their nature.

In my nursing practice I have always assumed that there is, indeed, this drive toward order and wholeness within each person. Within this context, professional nursing is one means of facilitating this natural process. It is an act of cooperation with the forces of nature; it is, essentially, an act of cultivation.

In order to cultivate, or intervene therapeutically, it is necessary to have knowledge of the various laws governing human well-being, knowledge of the condition of each individual requiring assistance, and the wisdom and discretion to treat appropriately.

The process of nursing assessment—the gaining of knowledge of the individual's condition—is thus a key aspect of the practice of nursing. If our knowledge of a particular client is erroneous or sketchy, all our good intentions and nursing theories will be of limited effectiveness. If, on the other hand, the data on the client have been carefully obtained in a thorough and reliable manner, we will be able to effectively utilize for this individual our store of knowledge about the healing process.

Assessing the Individual as a Unified Whole

Within a holistic perspective, nursing assessment is much more than a description of the client's physical state. Holistic assessment is an evaluation of the individual's total state of being. It is, moreover, an ongoing process, reflecting the changes that continually occur in human life.

A thorough assessment includes all the various aspects of humanness. For example, a human being has a physical aspect, so we can note such such things as the quality of his heartbeat and his gait, posture, and facial expressions. A person's facial expression very often gives us clues to his emotional state, another important component of our assessment. We must also try to discover the various ideas the client has about himself. For example, does he think of himself as basically healthy or as basically ill? And what is the client's spiritual state? Does life have significant meaning for the client? What are his beliefs about God, nature, life, and death? As discussed above, a human being is an integral part of the universe. He does not exist in a vacuum, so we therefore must obtain information about his environment (*i.e.*, his job, his school, his family, his friends, his daily habits).

After we have spent some time with our client, we will come away with a great many facts and observations. All of these are important, but not in isolation. Each element is a fragment of a magnificent pattern that must be placed in proper perspective so that the whole may emerge.

Quinn has emphasized the fact that assessment is not one isolated event but a continual process:[2]

> The nurse does not "do" an assessment once but uses each encounter with the client to gather new information, to clarify previously learned information, or to validate conclusions about the data already collected. Much can be learned about a client in a 5-minute interaction if the nurse uses that time well.

For example, suppose a girl named Suzie is admitted to our ward with a medical diagnosis of pneumonia. As we walk into Suzie's room, we see a heavy, dark-haired girl about 13 years of age. Her face is flushed and she has a dry, harsh cough. There is a feeling of "static" in the room. Suzie's mother tells us immediately that her daughter is a straight-A student and that the wall lamp is not bright enough for her to read.

As you can see, in less than a minute we have begun to pick up valuable information about Suzie and her environment. Suzie is obviously overweight and has a respiratory problem, so we must assess her physical needs very carefully. The feeling of static in the room and the mother's forceful manner give a clue that perhaps there is some emotional tension in the mother–daughter relationship that should be explored. As a young adolescent, Suzie's body image and sense of selfhood are most probably undergoing radical changes, so these elements should also be included in our assessment. It will be important for us to gradually uncover the meaning of the emphasis on straight A's. Is this Suzie's way of gaining her mother's approval? Is it her way of bolstering her own sense of self-worth during a difficult time? Does she have to study excessively to achieve these grades? Does she get some physical exercise every day? What kind of food is she eating? Does she have a boyfriend? A sense of humor?

We will find, during the assessment process, that all these aspects of Suzie's nature are interrelated. For example, if Suzie is under constant pressure to maintain an excellent scholastic average she might try to ease some of the tension by eating. The resulting obesity would most probably put a strain on her body image and peer relationships. To increase her self-esteem, she might turn away from the activities of her peer group and devote even more time to her studies. The lack of normal social activity would create additional stress for the young girl. Since stress is known to interfere with the functioning of the immune system, pneumonia would fit right into this pattern.

In a holistic assessment, it is this overall pattern of interrelationships rather than any one isolated piece of data that is meaningful. A physical symptom is often only the outward manifestation of a complex, multidimensional problem. Therefore, in seeking to understand our client, we must assess all aspects of his or her human nature.

Assessment as an Interaction

When we assess holistically, the major tools we use are ourselves. There is no machine on the market that will assess a client in a multidimensional manner. There are some very helpful assessment guides, such as the one developed by Quinn,[2] but we still must use ourselves to establish rapport with the clients; we must ask appropriate questions, make knowledgeable observations, and synthesize all the data into a meaningful pattern.

The assessment process is thus an interaction between two individuals. I, a human being, must use myself to evaluate another human being. My assessments, therefore, are a reflection not only of the client, but also of me. They reveal my knowledge, my clinical and interpersonal skills, my system of beliefs, values, attitudes, and the degree of rapport I am able to establish with the client.

For example, in order to fully appreciate Suzie's condition, I should have some knowledge about the nature of stress, infectious processes, human growth and development, family dynamics, and so on. The more extensive my knowledge and experience, the richer will be the patterns of my assessments. Also, the deeper the rapport that I establish with the clients, the freer they will feel about disclosing themselves, and the more pertinent data I will obtain.

"Through a Glass Darkly"

It is extremely difficult to keep our personal beliefs, values, and prejudices from influencing our assessments. We all have our particular ways of viewing reality, of making sense of the world, which Wallace calls a "mazeway."[3] Wallace writes that the mazeway is "nature, society, culture, personality, and body image, as seen by one person." Our personal mazeways help us to function effectively in our particular segment of society. However, they can also become rigid, blinding us to other ways of looking at the world and limiting our capacity for understanding and empathy.

Belief systems, or mazeways, tend to be self-perpetuating. Our own way of looking at things generally becomes established in childhood. We have had it with us a long time and it feels comfortable, like an old shoe. Consciously or unconsciously, we tend to associate with people whose ways of looking at reality are similar to our own. We talk to them every day and thus reinforce these values and beliefs.

We also talk to ourselves. Our likes and dislikes, opinions and desires constantly revolve in our heads. Casteneda has emphasized the fact that we uphold and strengthen our beliefs through this continual "internal talk."[4] According to Walsh, our internal dialogue, old thoughts, and fantasies imprison us in a world of our own making.[5]

Thus, through external and internal talking, we maintain our established beliefs and prejudices and these, in turn, limit our awareness. Krishnamurti has written that the rigidity of our beliefs separates us from other people.[6] We understand them only from one point of view, which, naturally, is our own.

I feel that in order to assess holistically we have to remove the barriers of belief and prejudice that separate us from the clients. We must develop an attitude of openness, of attentive receptiveness; in other words, we must learn to listen. An oriental philosopher once wrote that to know a man is not to know his name but to know his melody. This beautiful statement gives a very clear insight into the nature of holistic assessment; we try to listen to the melody of the individual. To listen clearly means to stop talking, to transcend for the moment our personal mazeway, and to be open to another person.

Casteneda describes an exercise that I have found very helpful as a preparation for holistic assessment.[4] For 15 minutes every day, he had to practice sitting calmly with his eyes closed and listening intently to "the sounds of the world." If you do this exercise for 15 minutes, if you really keep your eyes closed and your attention focused on "the sounds of the world," you will realize how difficult it is to quiet the internal dialogue and attain a state of attentive receptiveness. It is not easy, but if you practice daily you will see that the effort is well repaid. You will notice a gradual change in the way you perceive the world, a widening of the mazeway, so to speak. The exercise has helped me personally to relax, to stop prejudging and classifying so much, and to appreciate more deeply the rich complexity of every human being.

The Intuitive Element

In Suzie's case, the "feeling of static" in the hospital room was an important element of the assessment. Do you think that a nonverbal "gut-feeling" such as this is appropriate in a professional nursing assessment? Our modern scientific method is based upon the laws of logic, so it is easily understandable why one must assess logically. But what about intuition? Is this a valid means of conscious knowing? I feel that the intuitive processes are not only valid, but are necessary for this type of assessment. Our challenge at the present time is to try and understand intuition so that we can utilize it more appropriately and effectively.

Ornstein carefully documented the existence of two major modes of human consciousness.[7] One mode is analytical, sequential, and verbal, and is associated with the left hemisphere in the brain; the other mode is holistic, spatial, and nonverbal, and is associated with the right hemisphere of the brain. According to Ornstein, another way to convey this dichotomy is to describe the differences between the "rational" and "intuitive" aspects of human beings. These are complementary modes of knowing and many great achievements in human history have arisen through a suitable integration of these two modes.

For example, Michael Polanyi, the eminent philosopher of science, writes that the process of scientific discovery consists not only of analytical, rational thinking, but also of a qualitative and undefinable process, similar to perception, whereby a scientist organizes isolated pieces of knowledge into a meaningful whole.[8] This is intuition, which Polanyi calls the *tacit dimension*. He describes the scientist as knowing more than he can verbalize. At critical periods, after much knowledgeable deliberation, this tacit knowledge effortlessly breaks through, and discovery is made.

The intuitive processes, therefore, are those by means of which we integrate diverse elements into a meaningful whole. We use intuition when we recognize patterns, when we appreciate painting, sculpture, and music. We also use intuition during a holistic assessment, when we pick up subtle cues and perceive the connections among the various aspects of the client's being.

Within the holistic framework, a human being is a dynamic network, a complex web of interrelationships. In order to assess a client within this framework, we must make use of a nonlinear, spatial, acausal mode of knowing. We should not disregard rational analysis but rather should put it in its proper perspective.

For example, if suddenly we get the idea that Suzie's obesity, her aggressive mother, her good grades, and her pneumonia are all interrelated in a pattern of stress, we should check this insight with our intellects. What does our accumulated knowledge tell us about stress? Is our insight about Suzie's condition congruent with this knowledge? If we teach Suzie some techniques of stress reduction, is there a change in the pattern of her life? We must constantly check, balance, and support our intuition by the complementary use of reason, logic, and knowledge.

The Inner Stillness

Polanyi describes intuition as a mysterious element which works in the depths of our being, arising into conscious awareness in the forms of hunches, feelings, sudden insights. Ornstein also wrote that, due to the emphasis on rational thought in our culture, the intuitive processes function largely in the subconscious. However, because intuition is vitally necessary during a holistic assessment, we must cultivate it within ourselves; we must build bridges, as it were, between our conscious and subconscious aspects.

I have found that one effective method of doing this is to practice being still. This does not mean just a physical stillness—it means an overall quietude of being. If we are always running around after this and that, if our emotions are in a turmoil, if our thoughts keep darting from one subject to another, then the subtle intuitive insights have a very difficult time reaching awareness. Only when our beings are still can we hear our own inner voice.

You might very well ask me "How can I possibly be still when I work nights in the surgical intensive care unit with little help?"

I know that it is difficult, especially in a modern hospital situation.

Fortunately, in every culture of the world, there are techniques that help people attain states of inner stillness and integration. Casteneda's listening exercise is one very fine example. Other examples can be found in the books by Ornstein,[7] White,[9] and Naranjo and Ornstein[10] (these are listed in the references). According to Naranjo, most of these exercises involve a focusing of attention, a "dwelling upon" something. They involve an effort to focus and still the mind.

The important thing is to pick out a technique that appeals to you and to practice it on a regular basis. After a while, you will begin to get a feeling for this state of inner stillness. With a little more practice, you will be so well acquainted with it that you can create it within yourself any time you want to, especially before and during each assessment.

If you like the listening exercise described above, you might want to experiment by sitting outside and focusing on some natural sound, such as the sound of the ocean or a brook or that of the wind in the trees or the birds' songs. When you get distracted and when your thoughts wander, gently bring yourself back to the sound.

Because as all aspects of a human being are interrelated, this focusing and quieting of our minds also result in a quieting of our emotions and physical processes. And, in this stillness, we can hear both the client and ourselves more clearly than ever before.

Summary

Within the holistic framework, a human being is a dynamic pattern of physical, emotional, mental, and spiritual processes. A thorough assessment is one in which we evaluate the client as a complex, multidimensional whole.

While assessing a client holistically we must use ourselves as the principle tool. Both our rational and our intuitive aspects are integral to this process. We, in our wholeness, assess another in his or her wholeness. The assessment is thus an interaction process, the outcome being a reflection of both the client and ourselves.

In order to interact deeply, we must learn to put aside beliefs and prejudices that restrict our awareness and separate us from the client. We must learn to be still and to listen without distortion—to hear, as it were, with the ear of the heart.

References

1. Progoff I: The Symbolic and the Real. New York, McGraw-Hill, 1963
2. Quinn J: A guide for assessment. In Kennedy MS, Pfeifer GM (eds): Current

Practice in Nursing Care of the Adult: Issues and Concepts. St Louis, CV Mosby, 1979

3. Wallace AFC: Revitalization movements. American Anthropologist 58:264–281, 1956

4. Casteneda C: A Separate Reality: Further Conversations with Don Juan. New York, Simon & Schuster, 1971

5. Walsh R: Initial meditative experiences: Part I. Journal of Transpersonal Psychology 9:151–192, 1977

6. Krishnamurti J: The First and Last Freedom. New York, Harper & Row, 1954

7. Ornstein R: The Psychology of Consciousness. New York, WH Freeman, 1972

8. Polanyi M: Personal Knowledge. New York, Harper & Row, 1958

9. White J (ed): What is Meditation? Garden City, Anchor Press/Doubleday, 1974

10. Naranjo C, Ornstein R: On the Psychology of Meditation. New York, Viking Press, 1971

12 Using Imagery to Assess Patient Response to Therapeutic Touch

Patricia Heidt

As a psychotherapist–nurse I have been interested in how my patients view their own abilities to help or heal themselves. Guiding them to understand the meaning of their symptoms and to listen to the "messages" they have for them in their own growth process has been one of my primary goals. Several years ago I became acquainted with the research on Image-Ca, a diagnostic tool developed by Achterberg and Lawlis for predicting patient prognosis in illness.[1] These two researchers indicated that there was a relationship between the symbols selected by cancer patients to represent their perceptions of the disease process and the psychologic functioning of the patients at that time.

At the same time, I was involved in learning about Therapeutic Touch and was interested in developing a tool to measure its effectiveness with patients. Jeanne Achterberg thought that the tool, Image-Ca, could be adapted for this use and offered me some suggestions for doing this.* I tested it on a number of patients who came to a summer workshop on Therapeutic Touch conducted by Dr. Dolores Krieger and Dora Kunz at Craryville, New York. In this chapter I present (1) a review of research on the rationale for using imagery in the assessment–treatment process, and (2) a description of one patient who received intervention by Therapeutic Touch and who volunteered to experiment with me in using this creative imagery tool.

Rationale

The term *creative imagery* as used here denotes a kind of visualization made up of imaginary images. The component parts are derived from images of past perceptions and recombined to form new concepts and

*I am especially grateful to Drs. Achterberg and Lawlis for the permission and helpful suggestions offered to me in adapting the original tool for use in this research.

fantasies.[2] In order for images to form it does not matter whether there is an actual stimulation of the retina or an internal stimulus. Perceived events are stored as memories in the cortex of the brain and are ready to be evoked by some new and closely similar experience.[3,4]

It is suggested that although the ability to regenerate and employ mental imagery varies among people, the potential to do so is probably universal. Under appropriate conditions of training and performance, it is likely that all persons can utilize imagery.[2,5,6] Sarbin argues that the continued use of imagery is encouraged by social circumstances which lend the quality of "approval."[7]

From the following discussion of the literature, it may be deduced that imagery promotes a state of relaxation in patients and serves as a "placebo" to stimulate wellness.

Imagery Promotes Relaxation

Research has created a substantial foundation for a more comprehensive understanding of the relationship between mind and body. A core assumption of such theory asserts that "man's symbolic activity, . . . influences organismic processes at all levels of organization down to the cellular level . . ."[8] Humans interact with their environment, in which thoughts, memories, imagery, and fantasy all affect homeostasis, adaptation, and health, and in turn are influenced by such stimuli.

In health care, the implication is that consciously or unconsciously perceived "stressors" alter homeostasis and impose adaptive bodily demands, often culminating in states of illness.[9] Clinical investigation indicates that mental activity, in the form of visualization, can effect changes in the body's physiology to change states of stress to relaxation, which allows the body's constricted activities to assume their normal self-regulatory functions.[10-12]

Asking patients to clearly visualize the part of the body that is to be influenced sets up a contact with that particular body part, and a supply of information about the degree of tension of the muscles or viscera comes to the conscious awareness of the individual. Green and Green explain that activity in the voluntary nervous system occurs in the normally conscious domain, whereas autonomic nervous activity (such as visceral, circulatory, glandular, and other basic processes) occurs involuntarily and unconsciously.[13] In order to come in contact with these body parts one must develop a "kind of awareness of normally unconscious events." Visualization is one way of reaching the unconscious processes.

If psychologic processes interact with natural physical processes producing states of discomfort, pain, or disease, then these same psychologic processes can be used by individuals to gain control of their body functions.[1] Imagery that encourages the individuals to relax parts of their bodies can alleviate or eliminate the anxiety accompanying body discomfort. In this state of relaxation, individuals are more likely to mobilize their own inner resources for healing by becoming more aware and in contact with their bodies.

Imagery as Placebo

The history of health care is replete with research that indicates that suggestions, images, drugs, and the therapeutic relationship itself have been accepted by the patient so as to simulate and facilitate intrinsic healing processes.[14-16]

According to Simonton and Simonton, spontaneous remissions or unexpectedly good responses in treatment of cancer patients have one factor in common: the patients' "visualizing themselves being well."[17]

When patients utilize a creative imagery exercise they temporarily suspend the ordinary linear type of thought in favor of a more primary process type of thinking. Reyher states that when the patient is assisted in making this shift from rationale, expressive thinking of the left-hemisphere brain activity to the synthesizing, receptive functioning of the right-hemisphere brain activity, patient "suggestibility" is enhanced.[18] At this time, the patient is more likely to incorporate the instructions of the attending therapist into his or her own internal framework.

The motor power of the imagination, or "suggestion" as it is referred to by Assagioli,[19] implies that "every image has in itself a motor drive." This concept that the imagined idea and the incipient movement are approximately the same thing was termed "ideo-motor action" by W. B. Carpenter, a psychologist, in 1852.[20] Jacobson demonstrated this in a series of laboratory experiments.[12] Measurements of neuromuscular states were recorded as subjects were asked to "imagine" performing a wide variety of activities. For example, a subject previously trained to relax imagined that he was lifting a 10-pound weight with one arm to which electrodes were attached. A summary of average results indicated that during imagination electrical fluctuations occurred in the biceps region of the arm which were absent during the period of relaxation. As subjects imagined performing activities, small but measurable amounts of electrical activity were observed and graphed.

A supporting concept to the above is that of "neuromotor enhancement." Rugg states that the initial minute muscular responses produced through imagery can be greatly increased by suggestion.[21] As a thought produces excitation, a series of suggestions may eventually produce contractions that spread from one specific nerve channel to other related ones. The tissues maintain a state of normal tension and remain alert and ready to function in response to suitable stimuli.

Achterberg and Lawlis maintain that imagery is the process

involved in transmitting to the patient the expectation regarding his or her ability to return to health.[1] The "placebo effect," or what the patient images ought to happen following treatment, directly guides disease progress and treatment outcome.

The Case Description

Procedures

The patient in this research is R.T., an intelligent, attractive woman 39 years of age. She describes her illness as cancer in a state of remission following a 6-month period of radiation and chemotherapy. This treatment had ended 11 months prior to her participation in this research.

The imagery tool used to assess the patient perceptions is a modification of Image.[1] In this protocol, R.T. listened to a 10-minute tape which assisted her to relax each part of her body and to visualize the illness and any treatment she was receiving. After this, she was instructed to draw what she had imagined. A structured interview followed in which the nurse–investigator and the patient explored the following: (1) describe how your disease looks in your mind's eye; (2) describe how you see your body helping it go away; (3) describe how your treatment is working to rid your body of disease.

The drawings and interview were scored on 12 dimensions using 5-point scales. Three dimensions pertained to the disease process: vividness, activity, and strength of the cancer cell. Five dimensions pertained to the body's defense against the cancer process: vividness, activity, and strength of the white blood cell; relative comparison of the number and size of the white blood cells to the cancer cells; and strength of the white blood cell. Two dimensions pertained to medical treatment: vividness and effectiveness of medical treatment. The last two dimensions pertained to general aspects: symbolism of the imagery and overall strength of imagery or emotional investment of the patient. Scoring for dimension 13 was omitted because the patient had not been using imagery as a treatment modality. Scoring for dimension 14 was omitted because of the relative inexperience of the investigator in collecting imagery data.[1]

The imagery protocol was administered by the investigator to R.T. on Day 1 and Day 9 during the time that the patient was receiving treatment by Therapeutic Touch. A follow-up assessment was made 3 days post-treatment, 2 weeks post-treatment, and 1 month post-treatment. The patient received Therapeutic Touch twice daily for approximately 8 to 10 minutes from a registered nurse who was taught by Krieger or Kunz to administer such intervention. The times for treatment were early morning and late afternoon.

Research on Therapeutic Touch indicates the potential of this intervention for eliciting a state of physiologic relaxation in the patient.[22] The healer, who is in a state of more optimal energy than the healee, intentionally directs these excess energies for the use of the ill person so that the healee's state of energy becomes more like that of the healer. The role of the healing person, who is visualized as an open system of flowing energy, is to assist the ill person to restore an open, flowing, balanced interaction with the environment.[23]

Drawings and Assessment Dialogues

The following dialogue between the Investigator (I) and R.T. describes Figure 12–1, the first drawing by R.T. on Day *1* of treatment by Therapeutic Touch.

I: Can you tell me how your disease looks in your mind's eye?

R.T.: I see cockroaches scurrying around. I spear one because he is out in dead center. The others are crawling under bushes and I only see their tails. I am not fast enough to get to them. My spear is 6 feet long so I don't have to get too close. They are dirty things. Although I want to kill them, I am ambivalent about it. Sometimes I have a spray gun, and I wait quietly for them to appear.

I: Is there any activity going on?

R.T.: The cancer cells are stray cells, unorganized and alone. There is a single one here and there. I see them moving about in circles, but they stop every once in a while. They hide from me, but they have to come out eventually.

I: How strong do you think they are?

R.T.: They are not so tough. Maybe 6 to 8 inches long, bigger than usual. They are evasive. If I could get to them I could kill them.

I: How do you see your body helping your disease go away?

R.T.: The white blood cells are sluggish and immobile. I am bigger than they are, but they go places I can't go. There is just one of me, with one spear. I am standing solid from the waist down; I can't seem to attack fast enough. It's like a Mexican standoff.

I: How much activity is going on here?

R.T.: I spear just one at a time. I can't move very fast. I need to find a way to lure them out because I am just waiting for them to appear. They are moving very fast, and I can't move fast.

I: How well do you see your body working to make it go away?

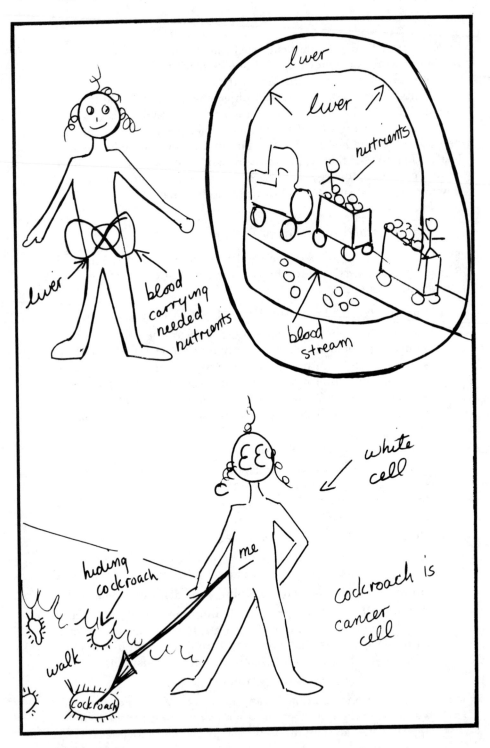

Figure 12–1.

R.T.: I see a figure eight of light in my liver—a bloodstream of nutrients. There is a train track going into the liver with two men on it. There is food on the cars and they are throwing it off. It is lying by the side of the tracks. This is to feed the liver. The train is moving slowly to the center of the liver. It comes back and gets a new load. If it can get to the center, it can be absorbed by the liver. The train is not getting to the center yet because they are still building the train tracks. There are people on each side putting braces along the walls and supporting the sides and roof of the tunnel. I guess . . . if the liver could work better, I can produce more little guys with spears to work for me . . .

I: How does your treatment work to rid your body of disease?

R.T.: The drugs are keeping the white blood cells down and this is not helpful. My white blood count is too low it seems to me. From February to April last year I had a raw food diet and my liver worked in top function and I bounced back quickly. I started to feel better and I then went back to my old diet of sweets and gained weight and am worse now. When I first heard I had cancer I said, "Well, my mother will be glad I am going to die."

I: How well do you see your treatment working to get rid of the disease?

R.T.: Well, there is obviously something I have got to get together. I can't afford analysis, but I might stop by and see my psychologist friend.

At the end of this dialogue, the Investigator asked for more clarification on the last statements, and focused on how the patient saw her relationship with her mother at the present time.

Figure 12–2 was drawn by the patient on Day 5 and given to the Investigator. There is no accompanying dialogue. It is part of the visualization used by the patient while receiving treatment by Therapeutic Touch.

The following dialogue describes Figure 12–3, the third drawing by R.T. on Day 9 of treatment by Therapeutic Touch.

I: How does your disease look in your mind's eye today?

R.T.: There is a brown crust of dead cockroaches surrounding the cabinet. I open the door. I have a shovel. It is hard work to loosen the crust. As a piece loosens it goes into the boiling acid. There are lots of dead roaches in that vat.

I: Is there any activity going on?

R.T.: There are two of us. You see this second person here in the drawing—very faint behind me. I don't know who it is. But there is a working relationship . . . a communication between us. The

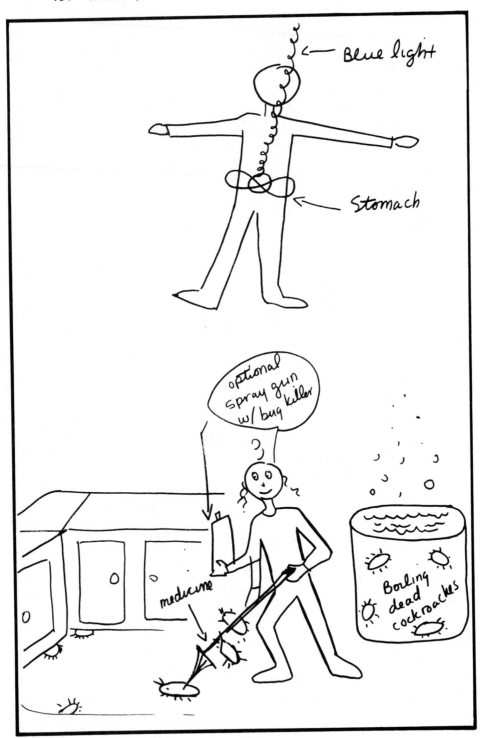

Figure 12-2.

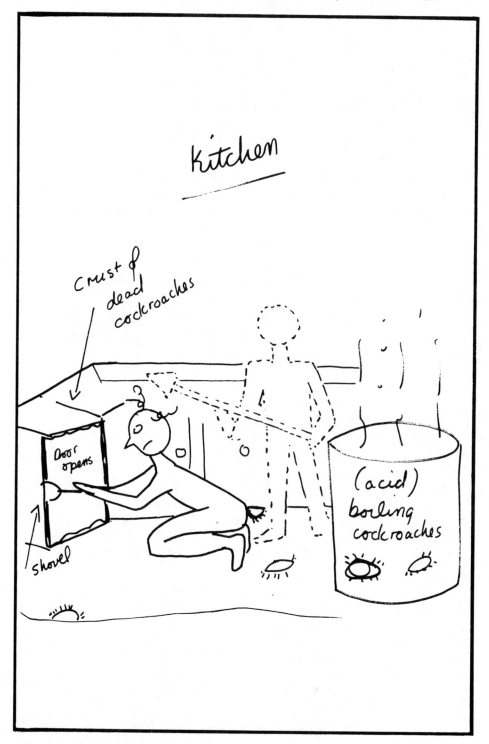

Figure 12–3.

more important job is now cleaning out the cabinets and I have gotten help.

I: How strong do you think the roaches are today?

R.T.: Well, there are many kitchen cabinets filled with dead crust. But I think there is a sense of purpose and order in my work. The person standing up there—the second person—is sort of ineffectual . . . The big job is inside the cabinets.

I: How do you see your body helping your disease go away?

R.T.: I'm not consistent at this. I do a little of the job at a time. Like I'm on the left wall and top of the back wall now. It needs to be done continuously . . .

I: How much activity is going on?

R.T.: Well, I am quite close to the cabinet you see. It looks like my arms are really bending and I'm in there swinging away, throwing those roaches into the vat.

I: How well do you see your body working to make it go away?

R.T.: Not too effectively yet. (*pause*) There is a conflict in my head. My superego says it has to get done right away. The child part of me says it will get done and at my own speed. Everything I did as a child was always wrong . . . But there is a strong voice coming through. I have got to trust it. It comes out in meditation times. When it comes through I know it is right.

I: How is your treatment working to rid your body of disease?

R.T.: I want to clean out that cabinet and make it stay clean. That's the next program in my fantasy work—I mean this physically and psychically. This is a crucial phase for me now. I want to focus not on the obvious cockroaches in the middle of the floor, but to get at the hidden stuff . . . (*pause*) The cockroaches are my illness, right? This is connected to my sadism. I need to get at the crust that is lining the cabinets. This is connected to years of hidden stuff . . .

At the end of this dialogue, the Investigator and the patient explored these last statements more fully, at which time the latter expressed her desire to return to psychotherapy for assistance.

Figures 12–4, 12–5, and 12–6 were sent to the Investigator by mail because the patient was interested in continuing the imaging process on her own following treatment.

The following comments accompany Figure 12–4, which was drawn 3 days post-treatment:

"After you and I talked about my going back to analysis for support in working with these images, the angel-like figure

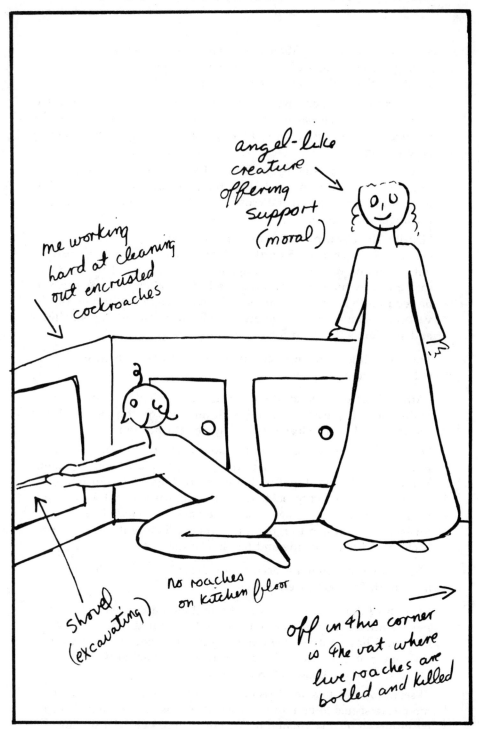

Figure 12–4.

appeared. I should say reappeared, because he used to be there during the last stages of my analysis in a supportive role. He speaks in the fantasy and encourages my work.

"I, the kneeling figure, work very hard at excavating the encrusted cockroaches in that particular kitchen cabinet. Sometimes I have to use heavy gardening gloves to tear parts away. Sometimes a shovel is sufficient.

"The image wasn't stable. Sometimes I would go back to it and find the crust had come back. Eventually, however, I stabilized the images and removed all the crust . . . with the encouragement of the angel-like figure.

"During the cleaning-out period, there were no (or only an occasional) roaches alive on the kitchen floor. I was able to deal with each one with the encouragement of the angel. I threw them into the vat which is at the other end of the kitchen. They seem to be reduced to a kind of compost which settles to the bottom of the vat and is somehow drained away. The vat is also getting smaller and smaller as the need for it seems to lessen."

The following comments accompany Figure 12–5, which was drawn 2 weeks post treatment:

"After I had removed all the crust in that particular cabinet, the white walls displeased me, and with the door on the cabinet, I was unsure whether if I closed it the crust might not re-form.

"So, in my fantasy, I removed the door permanently, and every now and again I check in there to see that no crust appears. Then, I crawled into the cabinet with a paintbrush and a can of white paint and proceeded to paint it with semigloss white. I wanted it to shine. Again, this image took some days to resolve. It was unstable. I often had to repaint and repaint before it 'took.' Now it is clean and white inside and has stayed that way."

The following comments accompany Figure 12–6, which was drawn 1 month following treatment:

"The third drawing is the current one. I am hard at work on the next cabinet. It is much more encrusted and filled than the last one and I have not yet been able to do much more than excavate the center of the crust. It keeps returning. The angel is still there offering encouragement . . . but less so.

"I seem to need less and less of his verbal encouragement, as the me-figure seems to be more motivated in this fantasy to finish the cleaning job in this kitchen to see how it looks clean. I see no more roaches on the floor, except an odd one here and there. Very seldom.

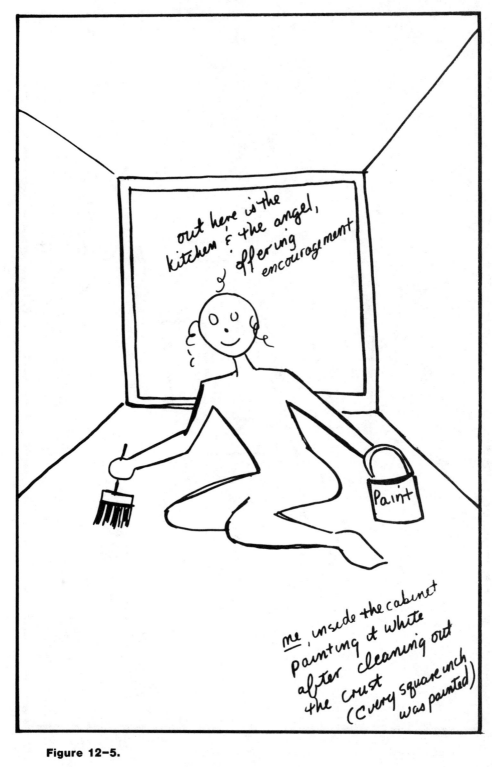

Figure 12-5.

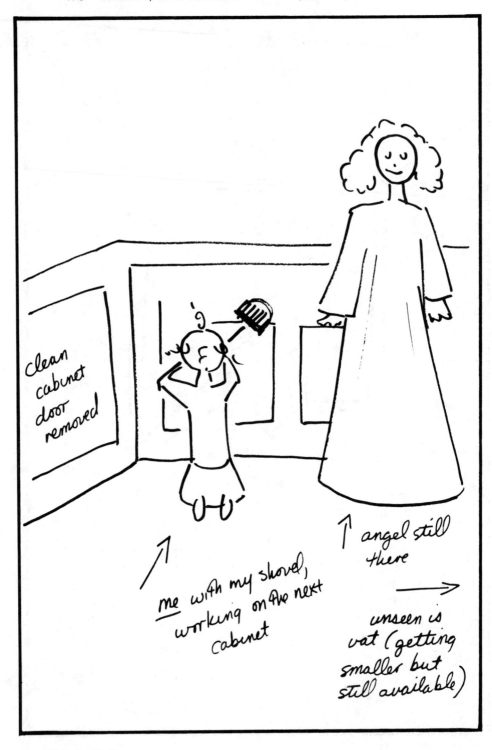

Figure 12-6.

"I have also removed the door from this cabinet. There are three more to do after I finish this one."

Analysis of Data and Discussion

The drawings and dialogues were scored by three judges independently. Based on 12 dimensions of the protocol, the imagery score for Day 1 averaged 91. The imagery score for Day 9 averaged 132. The primary shift in the difference in scores was in the area of the "Body's Defenses to the Disease Process."[1] The judges noted that the subject was able to imagine her body's defenses against the disease more vividly and actively. Also, the number, size, and strength of the cancer cells lessened in comparison to the strength and activity of the white blood cells. The overall strength of the imagery shifted from moderately weak to quite strong.

Because this is a case description of one subject, generalizations cannot be made from this data. Elsewhere I have attempted to make some generalizations based on further testing with similar subjects. It is interesting to note that in R.T.'s drawings and in the dialogues we both noted changes in her imagery as we discussed the data together. She noted that her cancer cells were first imagined as "something dirty" and that she wanted to hold them off at arm's length, using a long spear to get rid of them. She also indicated to me that she realized how tired she was in the dialogues: "I just can't attack fast enough"; and "The train is moving slowly . . ." I noted her response about her mother and asked her if she wanted to talk about this subject more.

As Figure 12–2 indicates, R.T. was treated several times daily during the workshop by Therapeutic Touch intervention, and was given a specific imagery exercise by Dora Kuntz to stimulate her own healing. This consisted of imaging a blue light descending into her body through her solar plexus area. When we discussed her drawings and dialogues on Day 9 together, she was pleased that she could note a calmness and a sense of purpose in what was happening to her. She remarked about her drawing: "Look at the change in my body—I am much more involved in what has to be done." I noted that she sees a relationship between her present symptoms and the long-standing "hidden stuff" which underlies her ability to get well.

Working with R.T. during this experimental period was very gratifying. She liked drawing these pictures and telling me about them. I sensed that it was very important for her to help me understand how she saw her illness in her overall life experience. She liked being able to use the treatment imagery and Therapeutic Touch interventions to stimulate her own healing processes. Equally important, she was glad she could talk about this very important process that was taking place within her and receive verification about it from me. In a way we became therapeutic partners in her getting well. I realized once again that as the patients become involved in their own assessment and treatment programs, they get to know themselves better. Illness, in these circumstances, becomes an opportunity for self-growth and self-renewal.

Experiential Exercise

1. With a friend, explore your own checklist for positive wellness.

2. Explore the use of imagery in your own life. You may wish to do this exercise with a friend or associate. (1) Spend some time relaxing and imagining each part of your body; think about any area of discomfort you are having and visualize your body getting rid of that pain; (2) draw what you imagined in any way you want, and, if possible, share your thoughts with this friend; (3) repeat this process in 2 weeks, and notice any differences in your feelings.

3. Have a conversation with a patient, a friend, a family member. Listen carefully to the number of times that they indicate feelings of helplessness about their own abilities to change their circumstances in life; notice the number of positive feelings, indicating a responsible and active participation in their attitudes toward their lives. Do not try to do anything, but listen carefully.

References

1. Achterberg J, Lawlis GF: Imagery of Cancer. Champaign, Institute for Personality and Ability Testing, 1978
2. Richardson M: Mental Imagery. London, Routledge and Kegan Paul, 1969
3. Eccles JC: Facing Reality. New York, Springer-Verlag, 1970
4. Neisser V: The processes of vision. In Richardson A (ed): Perception, Mechanism and Models. San Francisco, WH Freeman, 1972
5. Marks DF: Individual differences in the vividness of visual imagery and their effect on function. In Sheehan PW (ed): Function and Nature of Imagery, pp 234–249. New York, Academic Press, 1972
6. McKellar P: Imagination and Thinking. New York, Basic Books, 1957.
7. Sarbin T: Imaging as muted role-taking: a historical-linguistic analysis. In Sheehan PW (ed): Function and Nature of Imagery, pp 333–354. New York, Academic Press, 1972
8. Lipowski ZJ: Psychosomatic medicine in the seventies: an overview. The American Journal of Psychiatry 134, No. 3:233–245, 1977
9. Selye H: Stress Without Distress. New York, JB Lippincott, 1974
10. Luthe W: Autogenic training: method, research and application in medicine. American Journal of Psychotherapy 17:174–195, 1963

11. Wolpe J: Psychotherapy by Reciprocal Inhibition. Stanford, Stanford University Press, 1958
12. Jacobson E: Progressive Relaxation. Chicago, University of Chicago Press, 1938
13. Green E, Green A: Beyond Biofeedback. San Francisco, Delacourte Press, 1977
14. Torrey EF: The Mind Game: Witchdoctors and Psychiatrists. New York, Emerson Hall, 1972
15. Frank J: Persuasion and Healing. Baltimore, Johns Hopkins Press, 1961
16. Shapiro AK: The placebo effect in the history of medical treatment: implications for psychiatry. American Journal of Psychiatry 116:298–304, 1959
17. Simonton OC, Simonton S: Belief systems and the management of the emotional aspects of malignancy. Journal of Transpersonal Psychology 7:29–47, 1975
18. Reyher J; Spontaneous visual imagery: implications for psychoanalysis, psychopathology, and psychotherapy. Journal of Mental Imagery 2:253–274, 1977
19. Assagioli R: Psychosynthesis. New York, Viking Press, 1971
20. Eysenck HJ, Furneaux WD: Primary and secondary suggestibility. Journal of Experimental Psychology 35:485–503, 1945
21. Rugg H: Imagination. New York, Harper Row, 1963
22. Krieger D, Peper E, Ancoli S: Therapeutic touch: Searching for evidence of physiological change. Am J Nurs 79, No. 4:66–662, 1979
23. Krieger D: Healing by the laying-on of hands as a facilitator of bioenergetic change. The response in in-vivo human hemoglobin. International Journal of Psychoenergetic Systems 1:121–126, 1976
24. Heidt P: Assessment of the effects of therapeutic touch on patients' attitudes through use of imagery techniques. In Borelli M, Heidt P (eds): Readings in Therapeutic Touch. New York, Springer, 1980.

13 Stress Management as a Path Toward Wholeness

Lynn Wilson Brallier

Holistic Health and Stress Management

People in all cultures throughout recorded time have had to deal with stress. Many factors, including the prevailing philosophy or religious beliefs of a culture, have interplayed in the development of methods of managing stress. In the history of health care in the United States, we can see shifts in attitudes toward stress illnesses and in the ways that the health care industry has responded to helping people cope with stress. Prior to the era of specialization, country doctors or lay healers in the community cared for people as they attempted to cope with stressful life events or with stress that was of genetic origin or born of peoples' intrapsychic struggles. These helpers were often able to utilize a holistic approach when dealing with a person in distress because they knew the client's personality, social situation, work situation, family life, belief system, and general physical condition. However, the age of health care specialization ushered in a more technological and less humanistic and comprehensive approach to helping people manage their dysfunctional reactions to stress. This situation has often led to fragmented treatment, which may or may not be effective in relieving symptoms of distress. The modern treatment philosophy which views a person as analogous to a motor vehicle and proceeds to "fix" one part or another does not usually allow a person to learn how to avoid creating similar symptoms in the future and does not help a person examine and use his or her experience of illness as a step in growth toward wholeness.

The contemporary holistic health movement embraces principles of humanistic psychology. This fits together perfectly with the knowledge that in order to be of significant and long-lasting help to someone who is dealing with a stress-induced or stress-related illness, one must be aware of the nature of that person's body, mind, spirit, and environment. One must know how these parts of the person have interacted to create the distress. Psychophysiologic medicine, upon which much stress theory is based, has long paid attention to the interaction of body and mind. Emphasis in the past has been on how the mind has made the body ill. The holistic approach to stress management acknowledges this kind of interaction as valid and also helps people learn how their minds can heal their bodies. This approach also teaches people how to focus their minds in ways that help prevent their bodies from becoming so tense and distressed as to begin showing symptoms of disease. In a holistic approach to stress management, great emphasis is placed on the individual's responsibility for his or her own state of health. That is, the locus of control over one's health is within one's self. An educational approach to stress management is favored so that the individual can see himself or herself as a student who is reeducating or retraining his or her body to respond in a way that counters exaggerated forms of the body's distress response.

Use of the word "stress" in health care literature has been confusing because the term indicates both the cause and the result of trouble. For example, we say that stress is a factor in causing a heart attack and we also say that the heart attack itself is the stress. For the purposes of this discussion, we will use Hans Selye's definition of stress, which is that stress is "the nonspecific response of the body to any demand made upon it." Selye also defines "eustress" and "distress." *Eustress* is the body's response to a happy or pleasantly exciting event. *Distress* is a condition which comes about when someone is unhappy, frightened, or angry, or in some way unpleasantly excited. Besides these definitions of stress, it is important to recognize that there are both positive and negative effects of stress. The positive effects result from the fact that stress provides challenges for us, keeps us alert and interested in life, and occasionally stimulates large steps in personal growth and development. The negative effects of stress are experienced as unpleasant states of mind and body, usually having to do with a sense of being overwhelmed and not in full control of some aspect of life.

Another highly important aspect to know about stress is that stressors come in many forms. Varied events, ranging from a physical strain such as jogging or being physically injured to emotional strain such as hearing of the death of someone close or thinking a severely self-critical thought, can trigger a nonspecific bodily stress response. It is important to recognize that our own thoughts are a major source of stress for us. Ellis and Harper, in their writings on rational–emotive psychotherapy, have shown that many thoughts lead to arousal of the hypothalamus which is the center of emotions and influences the autonomic nervous system. Thoughts can be habitual and out of our awareness. They stem from what we were taught very early in life and also from our philosophy of life, our beliefs, and our attitudes. Thus, our storehouse of conditioned thoughts and thoughts stemming from our values have a significant influence on our level of distress.

Psychophysiology of Stress Responses

Hans Selye, who has probably contributed more research-based knowledge on stress than any other person in history, discovered a generalized response to stressors of all kinds which he calls the *General Adaptation Syndrome.*[2] This syndrome is generalized because it involves the autonomic nervous system and the endocrine glands of the body. The General Adaptation Syndrome is apparently an adaptive attempt by the body to deal with stressors while keeping the body in a homeostatic state. Selye uses the word *syndrome* because the body's reaction to stressors, no matter what their nature, is a rather orderly process with detectable stages. The exact nature of the General Adaptation Syndrome varies somewhat among individuals and also from one instance of stress to another owing to the presence of what Selye calls *conditioning factors.* These mediating conditioning factors may be genetically determined or they may be acquired.

The three stages of the General Adaptation Syndrome are (1) the stage in which there is an alarm reaction, (2) the stage of resistance, and (3) the stage of exhaustion. In other words, we may be somewhat shocked or alarmed by a stressor and at that time our nervous system and endocrine glands react quickly and predictably. If we survive the shock or alarm stage, we progress to the stage of resistance in which adaptation energy is utilized to cope with the stressor by returning the body to its normal homeostatic state. As exposure to the same stressor continues, our bodies enter a stage of exhaustion. Eventually, either our energy is depleted and death ensues or we replenish our energy and rebalance until the next stressor appears or is sought out.

Figure 13–1 illustrates what is presently known about the steps involved in a generalized response to a stressor. This illustration is extreme in its simplicity but serves as a tool for basic understanding of this response. As can be seen on the diagram, the stressor stimulates the hypothalamus, which then activates both the anterior pituitary gland and the autonomic nervous system, causing the latter to release adrenaline and noradrenaline. The anterior pituitary gland releases two hormones. One is adrenocorticotropic hormone, or ACTH, which travels by way of the bloostream to the adrenal cortex and helps signal this part of the adrenal gland to release syntoxic steroids or anti-inflammatory hormones such as cortisone. The other hormone released by the anterior pituitary is called somatotropin, or STH, which, in turn, stimulates the adrenal cortex and seems to cause the release of catatoxic steroids, or steroids which encourage an inflammatory response, such as aldosterone.

As was stated earlier, the General Adaptation Syndrome is apparently intended to help the organism maintain or quickly return to a homeostatic or balanced physiologic state. Under certain conditions,

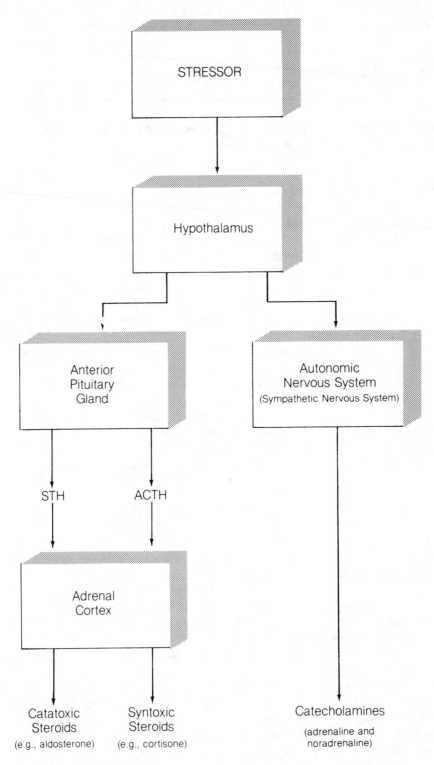

Figure 13-1.
The typical generalized response to a stressor.

such as when stressors are too intense or too frequent for the person to cope with, the body is unable to continue to effectively return to a normal state and a disease process is then likely to develop. For instance, too frequent an increase in the level of corticoids in the blood and in stimulation of the autonomic nervous system frequently creates peptic ulcers in the stomach and intestine. The corticoids also elicit thymus shrinkage and atrophy of lymph nodes as well as inhibition of inflammatory reactions. If all of these conditions become a chronic body state, a general depression of the efficacy of the immune system can result. This state of the immune system leaves a person vulnerable to many infectious diseases, probably including some types of viral cancers. Stressors, besides eliciting the General Adaptation Syndrome, can also influence the level of muscle tension in both striated and smooth muscles. This tension can eventually lead to problems such as tension headaches, back and neck pain, bruxism, and general pain and fatigue caused by muscles that are held in a chronic spastic state. Other typical stress responses involve the cardiovascular system and include hypertension, various forms of heart disease, strokes, and, in many cases, migraine headaches. Many allergic disorders may be seen as dysfunctional ways of coping with stressors.

Inability to cope well with stressors may also lead to accidents. Data from the field of biofeedback and from other relaxation therapies are making more clear the evidence that stressors are either causative or intimately related to nearly all nongenetically produced alteration in body structure and functioning. These data indicate that improvement or even cure of many disease processes can be brought about when a client is helped to learn a generalized relaxation response which seems to counter maladaptive features of the General Adaptation Syndrome. Clients with such illnesses as Raynaud's disease, Buerger's disease, and some forms of cancer—diseases that do not seem to be directly related to stressors—have shown remarkable improvement or remission when careful stress management and relaxation therapy have been utilized.

Evaluating Stressors and Their Effects

The first step in helping clients manage stressors so that they serve as challenges and motivating factors in their lives but do not lead to disease processes is to thoroughly evaluate past and present stressors and the stressors' effects on clients' bodies. Table 13–1 shows the Holmes and Rahe Social Readjustment Rating Scale. You may want to take a few moments to mark down your score for each life event according to whether or not the item applies to you in the past twelve months. For instance, if you have become divorced in the past twelve

Table 13–1.
The Holmes and Rahe Social Readjustment Rating Scale

Score Yourself on the Life Change Test

If any of these events have happened to you in the last 12 months, enter the Item Value in your score column. The items are listed so that the most stressful situation is at the top and the least stressful situation is at the bottom.

Item Value	Your Score	Life Event
100	_____	Death of spouse
73	_____	Divorce
65	_____	Marital separation
63	_____	Jail term
63	_____	Death of close family member
53	_____	Personal injury or illness
50	_____	Marriage
47	_____	Fired from job
45	_____	Marital reconciliation
45	_____	Retirement
44	_____	Change in health of family member
40	_____	Pregnancy
39	_____	Sex difficulties
39	_____	Gain new family member
39	_____	Business readjustment
38	_____	Change in financial state
37	_____	Death of close friend
36	_____	Change to different line of work
35	_____	Change in number of arguments with spouse
31	_____	Mortgage over $10,000
30	_____	Foreclosure of mortgage or loan
29	_____	Change in responsibilities at work
29	_____	Son or daughter leaving home
29	_____	Trouble with in-laws
28	_____	Outstanding personal achievement
26	_____	Spouse begins or stops work
26	_____	Begin or end school
24	_____	Revision of personal habits
23	_____	Trouble with boss
20	_____	Change in work hours or conditions

Item Value	Your Score	Life Event
20	_____	Change in residence
20	_____	Change in schools
19	_____	Change in recreation
19	_____	Change in church activities
18	_____	Change in social activities
17	_____	Mortgage or loan less than $10,000
16	_____	Change in sleeping habits
15	_____	Change in number of family get-togethers
15	_____	Change in eating habits
13	_____	Vacation
12	_____	Christmas
11	_____	Minor violations of the law
Total score for 12 months	_____	

Note: The more change you have, the more likely you are to get sick. Of those people with over 300 Life Change Units (your score) for the past year, almost 80% will get sick in the near future; with 150 to 299 Life Change Units, about 50% will get sick in the near future; with less than 150 Life Change Units, only about 30% will get sick in the near future.
(From the Journal of Psychosomatic Research 11:213–218, 1967)

months, in the second colum of the table you would write the number 73 on the second blank from the top. When you are finished, total the numbers you have written in and this will be your Life Change Score for the past twelve months. If your score is over 300, you have approximately a 90% chance of a very serious health change in the next two years. A score of 150 to 299 indicates approximately a 50% chance of a serious illness, and a score of less than 150 Life Change Units is correlated with a 30% chance of serious illness.

Figure 13–2 illustrates a rather casual but graphic method of determining your present patterns of exchanging energy with your environment as a way of measuring possible depletion of energy as a stress factor. In using this tool, begin by drawing a figure in the middle of a sheet of paper which symbolizes yourself. Add to that picture symbols that have meaning to you as representing people or activities that play an important part in your present life situation. Label each symbol as you draw it. Then draw arrows to and from yourself and each of the other people or activities in your picture. Let each arrow stand for one unit of energy. In some instances the energy exchange between you and another person or an activity may be equal; that is, you feel that you give as much energy as you get. In other instances, you may give two units of energy and receive only one in return and would

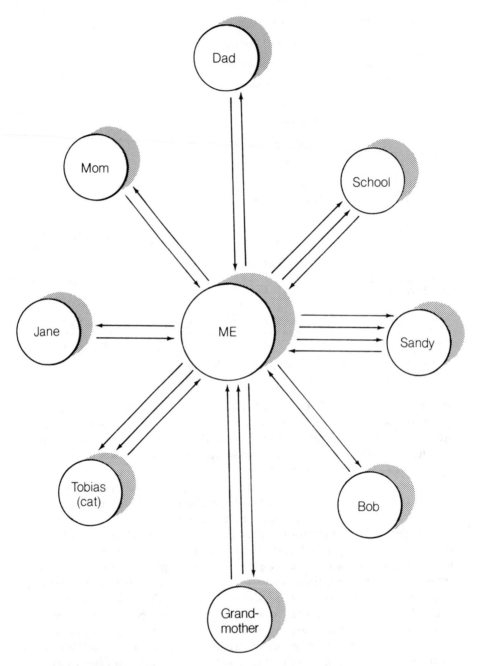

Figure 13–2.
The energy exchange stress evaluation drawing. (Stress Management Center of Metropolitan Washington, 621 Maryland Avenue, N.E., Washington, D.C. 20002. Used with permission.)

indicate that by two arrows going from you and one arrow coming back. When you are finished drawing in all the arrows, count the total number that are going out from you and the total that are coming toward you. Compare these two totals to see what the net result is in terms of energy exchange. If there are what seem to you to be a significantly higher number of arrows going out from you than toward you, you may want to consider the idea that you are stressing yourself by depleting your own life energy. A close look at this energy-exchange picture you have drawn may give you some hints on how to avoid such depletion of energy in the future.

A third way to evaluate stressors and their effects is to help clients (and one's self, of course) be aware of thoughts, attitudes, values, and beliefs that are mediating conditioning factors in their stress responses. For instance, let us say that a person holds a belief, which is either in or out of his or her awareness, to the effect that strangers are likely to be dangerous. If the person holding this belief is driving alongside another car and the other car eases toward his or her car, that person may react with fury and an intense physiologic stress response and may even lose control over his or her own vehicle. Someone who believes that strangers are "regular" people would be likely to assume that the other driver is being careless but not intentionally harmful and would stay calm and blow the horn as a brief signal to warn the other driver. Trying to be aware of subtle thoughts, often of a disparaging nature to one's self, can be difficult. Beginning by recalling a stress response and then tracing back to what one was thinking, even in a subtle form, just prior to the stress reaction may be a helpful method to use.

Another method of evaluating your level of distress is to note signs of distress in your body. For instance, let yourself reexperience some highly stressful event for approximately one minute and notice during that time which areas of your body become most tense, which areas become cool; or which areas perspire or become overly dry. Noticing these details of your body's probably typical reaction to a stressful event will help you be aware of your own patterned responses to stressors and will give you some ideas about which parts of your body to maintain a closer awareness of in order to keep these areas relaxed rather than tensed.

Another simple indicator of distress in the body is the temperature of one's hands. Warm, dry hands are a sign of relaxation and parasympathetic nervous system activity. Cool or cold hands, presuming that one does not have a circulatory disease and does not reside near the North Pole, indicate a state of distress in which the sympathetic nervous system is active. Preparing the body for "fight or flight" activity demands that the blood supply be channeled away from the periphery of the body.

Methods of Managing Distress Reactions

As you have seen in the previous section on evaluating stressors and their effects on the individual, stressors converge from the past, from the present, and even from thoughts of the future, and are of physical and psychologic origins. Stressors also interact with each other, so that helping a client unravel various stressors in order to become clear about them and manage them in a way that allows both equanimity and growth can be very challenging to the stress-management professional. Certainly the stress syndrome is not something to be approached in a narrow, specialized manner. Following the model used in my clinical practice, this discussion of methods of managing stressors is from a holistic theoretical framework. Therefore, we will be looking at physical, psychologic, spiritual, and environmental methods of managing stress. For a more detailed description of the philosophy and conceptual framework of holistic health and stress management in nursing practice, the reader is referred to the articles "The Nurse as Holistic Health Practitioner" and "Holistic Health Practice—Expanding the Role of the Psychiatric–Mental Health Nurse."[3,4]

The basic goals of stress management therapy are (1) to help the client learn to elicit the relaxation response and (2) to help the client learn to exchange chronic stressful patterns of thought and behavior for ones which bring about peaceful and satisfying coping. Fortunately, there are many physical methods of eliciting the relaxation response although individuals vary widely in their ability to utilize any given method for this purpose. For instance, some people find that active participation in running, swimming, tennis, or sexual encounters elicits deep relaxation, whereas others find that therapeutic massage, biofeedback, meditation, or even daydreaming are methods of choice to combat stress. Still others watch their diet very carefully so that their bodies are not stressed by foods to which they are allergic or by too much sugar, too many preservatives, or too much in the way of stimulants, such as caffeine, nicotine, alcohol, or other drugs. Therapeutic Touch is another method that is often very helpful in eliciting the relaxation response. In the case of stress management, it is wise to become an expert at many of these activities so that a wide range of choices is possible.

Perhaps biofeedback is the best example of a deliberate attempt to counter the harmful side-effects of the stress response. Biofeedback provides a technological way to allow people to gain control over their own bodily functioning. For instance, an instrument measures muscle tension or the temperature of a finger and then feeds back this information about the body's status to the client in visual and auditory forms; the client then relaxes and uses passive volition and visualization as ways of influencing his or her muscle tension and hand temperature. When a client can "hear" his or her muscle tension, he or she is then able to learn to control the degree of muscle relaxation he or she wishes to acquire. The same is true of hand temperature. Deliberately relaxing and redistributing blood flow into the peripheral parts of the body, such as the hands and feet, and relaxing muscles are ways to initiate a relaxation response. This involves, with mediation through the hypothalamus, the deactivation of the sympathetic nervous system and activation of the parasympathethic nervous system. The "fight or flight" syndrome, which was set off in the body by the reaction to a stressor, is now countered directly by the relaxation response. Biofeedback methods which help people thoroughly learn the relaxation response include instructions in various ways of breathing so that the body is well-oxygenated and the muscles of respiration are relaxed; various forms of autosuggestion so that constant messages are given to the self to relax, be calm, be comfortable; and the use of visualization or visual imagery. Imagery, that is, seeing a picture in the mind's eye, appears to be a powerful method of directing the body with the mind. Throughout history, many theories and schools of self-healing have also taught visual imagery methods. Biofeedback readings often change significantly when a person is able to construct a clear visual image of himself or herself in a relaxed environment (such as at the seashore with the waves lapping rhythmically and the warm sun shining its relaxing and energizing rays on the muscles of the body). Imagery can also be symbolic. For instance, biofeedback readings will also change in a positive direction if clients are able to construct clear symbolic representations of relaxation, such as seeing a piece of spaghetti as very loose and flexible or a feather floating in the air as representations of their muscles relaxing or the whole body feeling relaxed and light. Home practice of biofeedback methods of eliciting the relaxation response include listening to relaxation tapes and practicing various forms of meditation.

Biofeedback and meditation, as well as psychotherapy, are excellent methods of aiding people who are in psychologic distress. Physical insult to the body may elicit the General Adaptation Syndrome, but, most often, stressors in our current culture are of a psychologic nature and can lead to very serious stress reactions and disease processes. Psychologic states such as anxiety states, depression and chronic frustration, fear, resentment, anger, and worry can all lead to a dysfunctional adaptive response which, in turn, leads to physical illness. Poor self-esteem is another cause of being vulnerable to maladaptive stress responses in a chronic way. Failure to grieve losses properly is another cause of chronic distress and physical ailments. Utilizing biofeedback and meditation as ways of training the mind and body to elicit the relaxation response at will often helps a person be able to think more clearly about his or her psychologic reactions to stressors. These reactions most often are due to traumatic experiences during one's lifetime which were not resolved and are continually activated by new similar situations. Mind and body then become habituated to reacting in a stressful manner before the event or person being reacted to can be seen with uncluttered vision.

A comprehensive way of practicing psychotherapy with people in psychologic distress is to pay attention to both the cognitive and emotional components of the stress reaction. It is important for a client to look at his or her cognitive processes or the way he or she thinks about problematic situations. Often chronic negative attitudes and beliefs are found which are held more out of habit than reason. When these are corrected and replaced by positive attitudes and beliefs, the number and intensity of stress reactions decrease significantly. Attitudes toward one's self are extremely important in managing stress well. Keeping one's expectations of one's self and others at a reasonable level is important, as is the ability to be flexible and objective about one's self in certain instances. Being clear on what one wants at any given time and being able to take assertive action toward getting what one wants are important skills to have so that one does not unwittingly assume a victim role or a role that is so passive as to lead to constant disappointment and consequent distress.

Emotionally speaking, it is important to be able to let go of negative emotions in some way rather than harboring these and causing one's self distress. For example, one may help a client let go of chronically dysfunctional emotional reactions by enabling the client to release the old emotions through crying, screaming, or even laughter. The ability to interact emotionally with other people, with genuine love and good will and without an inordinate amount of emotional dependence, is also very important. A fine sense of humor is often a good tool in handling emotional stressors, and it is also an indicator that a person is distress-free enough to see the humorous or positive side of life situations.

The spiritual aspects of managing stress are very important and often neglected. Spiritual refers to our ability to rise beyond psychologic maturity into a realm of sensing that allows us to connect with a strongly positive force. This force or energy helps us make contact with and more fully develop our courage, our ability to genuinely love, our wisdom, and our compassion. This transcendental experience has been known by many names throughout history. Perhaps the most common contemporary term for the part of one's self that is involved and being developed by this experience is the "higher self." Often people who have spent much of their lives in a chronically distressed state find that they have developed a fairly unconscious philosophy of life that either includes debilitating spiritual values or spiritual values that they have outgrown. Others who have suffered chronic disease may have never clearly formulated any spiritual values and may never have been clearly in touch with that part of themselves. These are the clients who report a sense of purposelessness in life, a sense of having no goals; and a sense of life being an "empty stage" or even a "bad joke." It is interesting that the process of being still and focusing one's mind in meditation is so often of great help to people who are out of touch with their own spiritual side. It seems that the silence and focusing of meditation allow not only the mind and body to experience the relaxation response, but also allow the person to go "deeper" into himself or herself to gather senses, ideas, and feelings in a new way for what his or her life is about. Since we all react from a stance or a philosophical position about life whether or not we have consciously formulated this, being clear about one's life philosophy and spiritual beliefs can often add a sturdiness or a reserve energy to one's mental and emotional states. This reserve energy provides more stamina and less vulnerability to intense or prolonged stressors.

In our contemporary society, each decade has led to a greater concern about the stress factors in our environment. Pollution, chemicals used for processing foods, noise, overcrowding, economic problems, and many other important conditions make our active and bountiful culture also a place of very high distress. Usually it is people who compose the most impactful parts of our environment, and therefore social stresses are included in this section of discussion. Most people who are distressed complain that either family or work situations are sources of great upheaval for them. In these instances, it is very important to throughly review with the client details of the social environment which is distressing. Often the discovery is made that clients are playing dysfunctional roles in these situations or are reacting habitually in a distressful way because they are unable to see how to change their part in some of the patterned interactions. Typically, either at home or at work, stressful situations develop around issues of power and influence, over issues of emotional closeness and distance, and over the distribution of work among the people involved. There can also be severe value system conflicts among people who have more than a healthy amount of negative attitudes about themselves and others and so tend to be defensive. Helping clients take responsibility for themselves and let go of trying to change others in the environment is often a step forward in stress reduction. Deciding whether or not to stay in each of these environments is also a helpful decision-making process.

Other aspects of the physical environment are perhaps more easily dealt with. For instance, the home and office may be assessed to see that the living space is actually comfortable and enhances relaxation. Perhaps more space is needed, or more calming colors are needed within that space. Perhaps more comfortable furniture, a reduction in noise, or an increase in ways to provide more physical safety would be significantly helpful. Sunlight, temperature, and ventilation are also important factors in encouraging the maintenance of a relaxation response rather than a stress response.

An Educational Model of Stress Management

Some years ago in my independent practice as a psychotherapist and biofeedback therapist, I noticed that I was repeatedly teaching clients stress-management skills. Attuned to the holistic health concepts of self-responsibility and learning self-help health skills for both self-treatment and preventive purposes, I decided that many of the basic stress-management skills I was teaching to clients individually could be taught in a short course to a small group. I opened this to the community in general, hoping to attract people who were essentially well and who wanted to learn stress-management skills to stay well. What I have found is a potpourri of people who range from those interested in prevention to those who are in a terminal phase of cancer and who want to learn to manage the tremendous amount of distress and pain which often accompanies that life situation.

The course I am describing is called "Stress Management and Meditation." It is a 4-session course of 2-hour meetings and is designed to integrate cognitive and experiential material. One of the major tools to help students learn to elicit the relaxation response is a cassette tape I recorded, called "Suggestions for General Relaxation." Each student is given a copy of this cassette and is instructed to listen to it several times each day as homework practice between classes. This tape is similar to many relaxation tapes that I had recorded for people in biofeedback therapy. It is designed to help people learn to relax while staying alert. In the course, many forms of relaxation and meditation are taught so that people are given a choice as to which forms of activity or focusing of the mind are most likely to elicit the relaxation response for them. Biofeedback readings are taken at the beginning of the first class and again at the end of the course so that students can actually see their progress in terms of a decrease in muscle tension and an increased ability to raise the skin temperature of the hands. Attitudes and belief systems are discussed, as well as philosophical and spiritual issues as they relate to stress management.

Other educational approaches to teaching stress-management methods have been workshops, lectures, and individual and group stress evaluations and referrals. In each of these formats, the goal of helping people learn as many ways as possible to deactivate the stress response, which involves the sympathetic nervous system, and activate the relaxation response, which involves the parasympathetic nervous system, is kept as a primary task.

Clinical Practice

The Use of Holistic Health and Stress-Management Frameworks

As we have seen, dealing with the concept of distress and how it manifests itself in people's lives is a very complicated picture. Not only is there a near-infinite number of possible stressors interacting with each other in complicated ways, but also there are an equal number of possible dysfunctional reactions to these stressors since besides the stereotypic stress response there are unique individual reactions as well. Clearly this situation calls for a holistic approach, and so stress management has become a large part of the clinical practice of holistic health. In its beginnings, holistic health was predominantly a model of wellness, and it continues to embrace the idea of helping people move in the direction of a very high level of wellness. Now the framework has also expanded to include treating the whole person when that person is ill. As we have seen, people are most often ill owing to stress-induced disease processes or accidents, so the holistic framework and stress management in its comprehensive sense are excellent mates.

There are certain aspects of human potential that can form a basis for a holistic philosophy of stress-management practice. The first aspect is that human beings move naturally toward a state of wellness of wholeness. When the clinical practitioner believes this about human beings, he or she can then see stressors as blocks that inhibit people from their natural movement toward wellness. In other words, the essence of the clinical work is to help remove the impediments, and there is no necessity to worry about what direction a client will move toward once he or she has mastered the unblocking process. Occasionally a client will give up one stressful situation and take up another as if to replace the first, but this is unusual. Even in instances, when the client is ready to let go of the replacement block or distress, he or she will move toward wellness rather toward illness.

A second important aspect of human potential is that human beings have a virtually unlimited capacity for self-awareness. This is indeed fortunate because it provides a continuous avenue for detecting distress at earlier and earlier stages and in various, even subtle, forms, so that it can be deactivated and replaced with a relaxation response.

Self-awareness allows choices. Once we are aware of a stressful situation, we then must choose whether to handle it so that we experience distress, experience no harmful stress, or experience eustress.

A third quality of human potential is that human beings are capable of taking responsibility for their healing and their health status. This is an aspect of humanness which the medical model has often not honored. Instead, a condescending relationship with patients has been set up. In working with clients from a holistic stress-management philosophy, I have often spontaneously been called "coach" by several clients, and I was pleased at their recognition of the guiding rather than dictating position I have taken with them. From this position, clients are free to take the majority of the responsibility for their own state of health by learning as much as they wish about the functioning of their bodies and minds, about the effects of distress, and about how to cope with these effects. They are then able to feel a great deal of respect for themselves and their achievements and at having mastered their own destinies.

The fourth aspect of human potential which is important in a holistic stress-management framework is that human beings have the ability to regulate the status of their own health. Research in the field of biofeedback has gathered convincing data on this aspect of human potential. These biofeedback research data are rapidly refuting the ideas of only a few years ago that there are many functions of our minds and bodies that we cannot control. It is now clear that we can learn to control an almost unlimited number of body functions. An exciting new area of research is that of consciousness research, which is investigating theories that are both ancient and new concerning the control we can demonstrate over our bodies and our minds by utilizing meditative and visual-imaging methods in directing our energy. Self-healing and the use of Therapeutic Touch with the intent to help or heal are examples of this ability to direct the mind's energy. In these instances, persons can learn to accurately assess health problems and direct energy in such a way as to relieve these problems or even resolve them.

Applications of Holistic Health and Stress-Management Theories

In the following section, clinical work with three clients suffering from serious stress illnesses will be presented. Caution has been taken to change some of the identifying data so that these clients' anonymity is preserved.

Anita.　Anita, age 54, has been referred by her neurologist and has a history of 18 years of migraine headaches. She has had several complete neurologic workups over the years, including a brain scan, and no organic findings have been discovered. Both Anita and her doctor are concerned about the serious side-effects of the massive amounts of a very strong pain medication she has been taking.

A 2-hour assessment interview is scheduled with Anita, and during that session information is gathered in such a way that a holistic approach to her stress management can begin. A fairly detailed history is taken of her ability to cope with stressors from childhood to the present. The history reveals patterns of high sensitivity to stressors in which she has many times tried to be a buffer between people or has habitually repressed her own hostility during stressful situations. She has tried very hard to please her husband, her children, and the extended family, as well as her friends. This pattern of trying to please people has, in Anita's case, been useful to her husband's career as a United States Senator because Anita has been a very able crowd-pleaser at fund-raisers and campaign dinners, during speeches, and in general public-relations appearances. Anita has devoted herself to her family and to her husband's career, but is now beginning a phase of distress because her two children are adolescents and discuss their plans for college in the near future. She is struggling with what role or roles she wants to play now that the most active period of motherhood is coming to an end, and she is finding herself becoming aware of feeling unfulfilled in her role as helper in her husband's career. Anita is a perfectionist and obsesses about the details of her life-role decisions. She feels uncertain whether she will make the "right decisions so that everyone is happy."

During the initial interview, Anita's nutritional status is checked and she answers questions about food allergies. Questions about exercise are met with groans because Anita does not like to exercise but does have some awareness of her need to begin an exercise program. A biofeedback evaluation is done and familiar results are found. Her hand temperature while at rest is 76.4°F and drops during situational stress. Her muscle tension at rest measures higher than normal and increases significantly during situational stress. These data lead to the conclusion that her headaches are a combination of migraine and tension headaches.

During the initial session Anita is started on a biofeedback hand-warming training program. This is done with many clients with various stress ailments because it elicits a general relaxation response. Hand-warming is a specific treatment for migraine headaches. First the client learns to warm his or her hands at will using the biofeedback instruments and then is able to do this anywhere at any time without use of the biofeedback equipment. The client is then helped to be more aware of the subtle onset signs of a headache, and when one of these signs is noticed, the client warms his or her hands very quickly into the 90°F range. In most instances, the headache is aborted at that point by a mechanism that is still not fully understood. Anita is given this information as well as some time to practice relaxation and hand-warming with the biofeedback instrument. She is also given the tape "Suggestions for General Relaxation" to take home with her and is instructed to practice with the tape between two to six times each day. A small thermometer is also sent home with Anita so that she can utilize a very simple but effective form of biofeedback in practicing her hand-warming methods.

During subsequent visits, Anita is taught how to use acupressure points to help relieve pain should she allow a headache to occur. She is also helped to pay more attention to a diet which was recommended to her by a nutritionist and which involves eliminating sugar and chocolate from her food intake and adding vitamin B and C supplements. For exercise, Anita is helped to decide to take a dance class so that exercising will not prove to be a boring, lonely endeavor. She is also referred to an excellent medical massage therapist for weekly massages with special attention to the upper back, neck, and scalp muscles.

After the biofeedback, massage therapy, nutritional program, and exercise program are established, psychotherapy is begun with Anita to help her become more assertive, to help her let go of her perfectionism, and to help her deal in depth with her distress about her goals in life and the meaning of her life. Some sessions for couples' therapy are initiated to help Anita and her husband sort out her new role in his career. Anita and her husband are able to redefine this new role in a satisfactory way. The redefinition includes sorting out which speaking engagements, public appearances, interviews, and other public contacts for her husband's political campaign are minimally necessary for Anita to fill. Anita's high motivation to be free of her headaches and to enjoy a finer quality of life is an asset to this holistic approach to her therapy, and she is able to complete her therapy in 8 months, becoming essentially headache-free. A 1-year follow-up report from Anita indicates that she has been able to follow her therapeutic regimen successfully and is feeling a high level of energy and wellness.

Susan. Susan is referred by her physician for stress-management therapy after she sees a television program about biofeedback and its use with Raynaud's disease. Susan suffers from Raynaud's disease secondary to lupus erythematosus. She is aware that her hands become a dusky bluish-black color and her fingers are in significant pain when she is in specific stressful situations. She is a housewife and the mother of four adolescents, and she is already in psychotherapy to handle the depression and distress that have accompanied her battle with lupus. Susan is a highly motivated client because she is faced with the possibility of having to have one or more of her fingers amputated should the circulation in the fingers become poor enough to cause a gangrenous condition. She and her husband have decided not to move to a warmer climate because they feel at home in the metropolitan area in which they live, and so she is excited to learn of a method of handling her reaction to stressors in her life that would help her substitute hand-warming and a general relaxation response for her typical distress responses.

Susan is advised to take the stress-management and meditation course since she is already in psychotherapy. She does this and practices with the "Suggestions for General Relaxation" tape 6 times each day. A hand-warming thermometer is sent home with her so that she can get feedback on the actual temperature rise in her hands as she learns to relax and warm her fingers. Susan's psychotherapist is amazed that Susan is willing to learn general relaxation along with the hand-warming because she has had difficulty convincing Susan to alter her schedule to allow relaxation time. Susan proves to be a real expert at warming her hands within a few days of practice and easily warms her hands into the 90°F range at will. She continues to work at developing a "warm hand consciousness," that is, being aware at some level of her consciousness to keep her hands warm while she's awake and to give herself strong suggestions before she goes to sleep that she will be able to maintain warmth in her hands during the night. Meanwhile, Susan's diet and exercise were investigated. Susan is already very careful of her diet and takes appropriate vitamin and mineral supplements. She was taught exercises that would energize her, tone her muscles, and improve her circulation without causing her more pain and distress, and she is able to continue with this program. After she completed the stress-management and meditation course, Susan decided to be seen once every 3 or 4 months for office visits as a way to keep her motivation high and to check in for any new methods she might learn to relax and maintain warmth in her fingers.

Jack. Jack is 42 years old. He was referred for stress-management therapy by his friend after he suffered his first heart attack. Jack is a very hard-working lobbyist, and he has been working as much as 18 to 20 hours a day when Congress is in session. He has been working for the same lobbying group for 12 years and has been in an intense pattern of competing with his boss and getting annoyed with his staff if they are not as quick and hard-working as he is. Because Jack is accustomed to being a high achiever, he also applies this personality trait to achieving well in his stress-management therapy.

A biofeedback evaluation indicates that Jack has extremely high muscle tension; work with the electromyograph biofeedback instrument begins immediately. Jack is given the "Suggestions for General Relaxation" tape to practice with at home and at work. True to his nature, Jack decides to run the show at work and manages to get the entire staff to listen with him to the relaxation tape during their lunch break. The results delight him and he claims that people are getting along with much less friction than before and that even he and his boss are less competitive and negative toward each other. Jack has been in a pattern of ignoring his fatigue and the biofeedback helps him to be more aware of his body and its needs for rest. He is able, because of his fear of another heart attack, to pay more attention to his body's signals for the need for relaxation, and he makes a significant change in his daily routine. Jack is also referred for massage therapy and finds these sessions extremely helpful to him for body relaxation and awareness as well as for learning more about how he can move his body in ways that will relieve muscle tension as it builds during the week.

Jack is already seeing a nutritionist for guidance and is in a cardiac rehabilitation program for constant monitoring and guidance of his exercise. He is an avid reader and is given a bibliography on stress management. He reports that he has learned a great deal from his reading. We also explore his attitudes and beliefs about working hard and high achievement and find that Jack is able to let go of some of his more strenuous goals for his career in favor of living a longer and higher-quality life.

Summary

As we have seen in this chapter, dysfunctional reactions to stressors in our lives are perhaps the major cause for illness and accidents. A clear trend is developing in the health professions to pay more attention to dysfunctional attempts to handle stressors. Fortunately, there are some rather uncomplicated ways of deactivating a distress response and substituting a general relaxation response. Many of these methods of stress management can be learned quickly and practiced outside the health-care setting, with the health-care professional taking a teaching and consultation role more than a direct care role with clients. Direct care roles, however, remain very important and include delivering the services of biofeedback, psychotherapy, massage therapy, acupressure therapy, and Therapeutic Touch. More than delivering the services, what seems to be important in helping people learn to cope with life stressors is the context of the helping relationship. Incorporating Therapeutic Touch into the practice of stress-management therapy allows a new dimension of the helping relationship to emerge. Teaching clients how to use Therapeutic Touch with their family members and friends is also a way to enrich the quality of life and reduce the experience of distress.

The implications of this new interest in stress and its management for professional education and clinical practice in nursing are many. These include the need to learn in detail the psychophysiology of responses to stress and the thousands of ways stress reactions can manifest themselves in people's lives. It is important to learn the major ways that have been shown to be helpful in managing stress as well as ways to help a person discover his or her own methods of managing stress. Being an expert in stress management is an important part of playing a successful professional role with clients. When one is able to deliberately evoke a relaxation response and experience a calming and healing silence in meditation, then one can be an expert teacher and consultant as well as a healer. No matter what specialty area of nursing is practiced, knowledge about stress and the ability to act as teacher and consultant to clients about their stress problems will be invaluable in the future.

References

1. Selye H: Stress Without Distress, p 14. New York, The New American Library, 1974
2. Selye H: The Stress of Life, 2nd ed, p 38. New York, McGraw-Hill, 1978
3. Brallier LW: The nurse as holistic health practitioner. Nurs Clin North Am 13, No. 4:643–655, 1976
4. Brallier LW: Holistic health practice—expanding the role of the psychiatric-mental health nurse. In Community Mental Health Nursing: an Ecological Perspective, pp 219–228. St Louis, CV Mosby, 1980

Suggested Readings

Ellis A, Harper R: A New Guide to Rational Living. North Hollywood, Wilshire Book Company, 1979

Pelletier KR: Mind as Healer, Mind as Slayer. New York, Delta Books, 1977

Simonton OC, Matthews-Simonton S, Creighton J: Getting Well Again. Los Angeles, J. P. Tarcher, 1978

14 Client Care and Nurse Involvement in a Holistic Framework

Janet F. Quinn

In the Rogerian conceptual system, a human being is defined as an energy field, an open system engaged in continual energy exchange with the environment.[1] By definition, an energy field is a nonphysical phenomenon. We know that an energy field exists only because we can observe some physical manifestation of that field and not because we can see the field itself. A perfect example is a magnetic field. Although we cannot directly observe this energy field, if we subject a cluster of iron filings to the influence of a magnet, we will observe that the randomness of their distribution disappears; there occurs a reordering, an organization of the iron filings into a distinctive pattern. In this instance, we are not observing the field directly, but we are quite certain that it exists because we can observe the pattern and organization of the iron filings, that is, the physical manifestation of the field.

Given this conceptualization of the human as an energy field, one must begin to look at the behaviors of humans in a different way. All of a person's behaviors are manifestations of the unique pattern and organization of the energy field which *is* that person. Health, illness, and healing are equal possible outcomes or manifestations of human–environment energy exchange. Simplistic models of wellness and illness based on cause and effect are not valid within this conceptual framework, thus necessitating a shift in our focus when examining these phenomena. We must begin to search for information about the pattern and organization of the energy field during periods of health and illness so that intervention may be geared toward healthful repatterning.

The Nursing Process Within a Holistic Framework

Yura and Walsh define the nursing process as "the designated series of actions intended to fulfill the purpose of nursing—to maintain the client's optimal wellness—and, if this state changes, to provide the amount and quality of nursing care his situation demands to direct him back to wellness."[2] The four phases of the nursing process delineated by these authors are (1) assessment, (2) planning, (3) implementation, and (4) evaluation. Since its introduction in the early 1970s, the nursing process has become a well-established model for providing patient care. Regardless of the conceptual framework to which one subscribes, the nursing process can be utilized in providing care within that framework. Let us now examine how a holistic conceptual framework may be utilized in each phase of the nursing process.

Assessment

During the assessment phase of the nursing process, data are collected about the client to determine actual or potential problems. Traditionally, we have been concerned with gathering information related to the biologic, psychologic, social, and cultural dimensions of the client in making these determinations. However, when practicing within a holistic framework, assessment must be broader and deeper than this, recognizing that the bio-psycho-socio-cultural behaviors of humans are inherently interdependent manifestations of the energy field.

Increasing the breadth of assessment involves analysis of the relationships that exist between and among the biologic, psychologic, social, and cultural data gathered about the client. The patterns manifested by whole man are not the result of the isolated activities of these sub-parts. Rather, they reflect the synthesis of many complex processes into an organized, synergistic whole. What happens in one dimension always influences and is influenced by what happens in all other dimensions. Thus, to obtain a more complete view of a client's holistic patterns, we must look for these relationships in the assessment data.

The depth of the client assessment can be increased as far as the sensitivity of the nurse permits. All of the data we need about a client are there; they are available and accessible to discovery through sensitive perceptivity on the part of the nurse. Remember that, ultimately, we are attempting to gain information about the pattern and organization of an energy field. At this time the best tool we have available for directly experiencing a human field is our own human field. When a nurse engages in an interaction from a centered, open, and other-directed state of being, his or her perceptivity to subtle field energies can be enhanced. Consider the following.

On my stereo tuner there is a switch labeled "mute." In the on position, this switch allows reception of only the very strongest, clearest radio signals, and completely eliminates static and noise while the tuning dial is turned. When the mute switch is not in operation, even the very weakest signals may be received, albeit with considerable noise and interference between the tuned stations. Thus, I am given a choice each time I turn on the tuner. I can choose to utilize the muting circuitry, which allows me to hear an adequate variety of programs with virtually no effort on my part, or I can choose to leave the mute switch in the off position. In the latter case, more effort is required of me in fine-tuning the stations, but the range of programs to which I then have access is significantly increased.

The situation just described is analogous to the assessment process in several ways. Many "signals" emanate from the client-field as the client interacts with the environment. Some of these signals are exceptionally strong and easily perceived by the nurse-field. For example, a person's general appearance, height, weight, hair color, and gait and most other observations that can be made relative to the biologic or physical dimension are relatively "strong signals." When the focus of assessment turns to the psychologic dimension, we are attempting to perceive signals of a somewhat weaker, subtler nature, and so greater sensitivity is required by the nurse. The *actual* pattern and organization of the client-field's energies may be thought of as the weakest, or subtlest, signals of all, in contrast to the stronger signals, which are *manifestations* of the field energies.

Bearing in mind the distinction between receiving and perceiving, we realize that the nurse, as receiver, will perceive only those signals to which he or she is sensitive. Just as the tuner is equipped to receive both strong and weak signals, the nurse-field *receives* all signals from the client-field during continual interaction of their respective fields. Most of us, however, operate with some sort of muting in terms of our perceptivity, and so our discernment is limited to the more easily perceived signals. One must remember that all of the client's "signals" are present all of the time, just as radio waves never cease to surround us. Therefore, we are limited only to the extent of our perceptivity and sensitivity; our willingness and ability to "tune in" these signals.

This sensitivity to the client at the subtlest, most intimate level is a matter in which we have some choice. We can literally choose to leave the muting switch off or on by consciously developing and expanding our own perceptivity in the former case or by accepting the limitations of our sensitivity as they are in the latter case.

It is exactly this openness and sensitivity to the energy field of the client which are utilized in the process of assessment during Therapeutic Touch (described elsewhere in this book). The nurse utilizes his or her hands in determining the pattern and organization of the client's energy field. Subtle changes in the constancy of energy distribution throughout the field are sought out, as are imbalances in the flow of energy. A "normal" or healthy field will feel consistent and symmetrically distributed. Differences in the "feel" of the field from one area of the physical body to another indicate energy patterns that may be less healthful.

While I have noted that the nurse utilizes his or her hands in doing an energy assessment, it should be borne in mind that the assessment is holistic in nature. The nurse as a whole energy field is engaged in the process. The hands of the nurse serve as a focal point of reference during the assessment; however, the information gleaned is perceived through the nurse's own energy field. Thus, a nurse may feel an area of localized heat when scanning the client with his or her hands, but the understanding of what that heat means, the perception, usually comes as a moment of insight in the consciousness of the nurse. Conversely, insights may arise within the perceptive nurse without the use of the hands at all. The key is the perceptivity of the nurse when interacting with clients; the antennae must be extended if the nurse is to perceive these subtle signals.

In assessing the energy patterns of a client, there is a wealth of information available to the nurse. One becomes acquainted with the client at a most intimate, holistic level, experiencing who the client really is in a beautifully direct way. Subtle feelings or conflicts of which even the client was not consciously aware may become evident. Areas of tension or pain within the physical body are easily discerned while assessing the energy field. This information, combined with the assessment data collected about the biologic, psychologic, social, and cultural dimensions of the client, provides the nurse with a rich and potent data base from which determinations of holistic patterns can be made.

Planning

Once the nurse has identified holistic patterns that are actually or potentially less healthful, a plan for intervention must be established. The goal of such intervention will be to assist the client in repatterning toward a higher level of wellness.

Remembering that all behaviors are manifestations of the energy field that is the client, the nurse will be careful not to limit the plan for intervention to only the symptoms of dis-ease within the field. Short-range goals for intervention may well have one or more particular manifestations of dis-ease as their focus, for no doubt these symptoms will be a source of greater or lesser discomfort to the client. However, long-range goals must also be esablished, with a focus on the holistic patterns of the client that have manifested as illness at this point in space and time. If these patterns remain unchanged, we have done little to assist the client in moving toward health, even if the actual symptoms of dis-ease and the current illness are resolved. In this case, we might expect the client to develop some new behavioral manifestation of dis-ease, and to again require restorative intervention.

Establishment of long-term goals must be done by the client, with the assistance of the nurse, if they are to be accomplished. It is the client who must repattern, and therefore it is the client who ultimately decides what patterns or behaviors he or she wishes to change, and when. Goals imposed from without seldom reach fulfillment; it is a sense of responsibility for self that must be cultivated in the client.

Implementation

In this age of modern technology, we are provided with a seemingly inexhaustible array of gadgets, machines, chemotherapeutic agents, and other tools for nursing intervention. All of these tools are useful, as far as they go, in aiding the client's movement toward wellness. Yet, there is another tool, one which we always have available. It requires no requisition and has, perhaps, the greatest potential for helping/healing. That tool is, of course, our own "self."

When the process of assessment was discussed earlier, a great deal of emphasis was placed on the sensitivity and perceptivity of the nurse in determining energy patterns. During the implementation phase of the nursing process, this same sensitivity comes into play. We can immediately think of therapeutic communication—listening to and talking with clients—as one example of the therapeutic use of self. Obviously, the more sensitive and empathetic the nurse, the more effective and therapeutic the communication.

Another example of the therapeutic use of self is the use of touch, which is a fundamental, inherent part of nursing care. Yet so often our touching of clients is an almost unconscious process, much like blinking or walking or driving a car. Even when we are attempting to support or comfort a client with touch, we can and often do remain unconnected to the intimacy of that act, to the dynamic exchange of energy which is taking place, literally, right under our noses.

All nursing interventions should be purposeful, and the use of touch is no exception. When nurses utilize touch in a conscious way, with the intention of helping or healing clients, and approach the act of touching from a centered, self-transcending perspective, they have at their disposal a powerful tool for holistic intervention.

The nurse may utilize touch to exchange or transfer energy to the client. This energy input may serve as a catalyst, a stimulant to the client's own recuperative potentials. Symptoms of dis-ease may be relieved as imbalances in the energy flow of the field are corrected, and the client is provided with energy to be utilized in repatterning of his or her energy field. This process is, of course, Therapeutic Touch, as developed by Dr. Krieger,[3] and it is an appropriate and useful supplement to other modalities for nursing intervention within a holistic framework.

Evaluation

In this final phase of the nursing process, we are concerned with making a determination about the effectiveness of our nursing intervention. Sometimes this determination is easier to make than at other times. When a goal for nursing intervention has been to maintain the integrity of the skin of a bed-ridden client, the judgment relative to the effectiveness of nursing actions taken toward that end is fairly uncomplicated; either the skin is intact or it isn't. But when we are concerned with the repatterning of the client's energy field, these judgments may not always be so readily made.

It must be remembered that we are working toward change at a very deep and subtle level, and so when we look for manifestations of change, we may not always see dramatic transitions. More often we might hope to see a higher level of awareness manifested by the client, an insight into the interconnectedness of all facets of his or her life, a realization that, for example, the client's job is literally making him or her sick. These insights or realizations are the stuff that change is made of and, if we have assisted clients to reach this new level of awareness, we have done much to facilitate the process of repatterning toward health.

If we remain open and perceptive during evaluation, we may also discern that, indeed, there is a difference at the deepest levels of the client's being. We feel differently in his or her presence—perhaps more relaxed, more hopeful, more whole. If we reassess the patterns of the energy field, we can discern the changes that have taken place. There may be a feeling of fullness where there was limpness, balance in place of asymmetry.

It is perhaps more important during this phase of the nursing process than any other for the nurse to remain nonjudgmental. Energy directed for the benefit of the client will be utilized in whatever way is best for that unique client-field, and therefore we cannot always know to what precise end the energy we provide will be utilized. Movement toward health, for example, may actually be manifested as acceptance of death with greater equanimity and peace, rather than by "curing" of the actual pathology.

The nurse must also be willing to confront and accept the limitations of human-field interaction. In some instances, despite a centered, open, caring, and perceptive posture on the part of the nurse, there simply won't seem to be any difference in the client-field. In evaluating the effectiveness of nursing intervention, the nurse will have to consider the intervention to have been ineffective. In an instance such as this, it is important to recognize that ultimate responsibility for change lies with the client. Sometimes a client is not yet able or willing to allow the nurse to help him or her, despite all appearances to the contrary. The nurse will need to accept this without being judgmental toward the client, and especially not being judgmental toward himself or herself.

Holistic Involvement With Clients: Therapeutic for Whom?

In the preceding discussion, we have seen how nursing may be practiced within a holistic conceptual framework, utilizing the nursing process as a guideline for the process of intervention. Interwoven throughout that discussion is the idea that in truly holistic nursing there is an involvement of the whole self that is nursing at a most profound level. There are undoubtedly those who consider such an intimate involvement to be beyond the scope of nursing practice, and in fact to be dangerous to the emotional well-being of the nurse. In the following discussion, we will see that involvement of this nature—a holistic involvement—is as beneficial and therapeutic for the nurse as it is for the client.

The Nature of Giving

Suppose that I have something which you want—an apple, let's say, for simplicity—and I suddenly realize that you are trying to take my apple. I may react by saying to myself: "Oh no, this is *my* apple and no one is going to take it from me." Perhaps then we might struggle; you may physically try to take the apple from my hand, and I will resist with whatever strength it takes. Regardless of who ends up with the apple, how do you suppose we will both feel at the end of the struggle? I think it is a safe assumption that some amount of exhaustion would follow such an encounter, accompanied by a variety of unpleasant and uncomfortable feelings for both of us.

Now consider another possible outcome for the same situation. I sense that you would like to have my apple, so I simply give it to you. There is no struggle; I give you the apple willingly and consciously, knowing that I can get another. How would we both feel at the end of this encounter? Instead of exhaustion and discomfort, we might feel refreshed and satisfied. I, as the giver, have expended very little of my own energy, and in fact feel more energized, having engaged in a giving exchange rather than a struggle.

The point of this anecdote is simply this: no one can *take* from you when you are *giving*. I am speaking now of a giving which comes from a very clear, very centered stance. We have all encountered people who give and give and give until there is virtually nothing left for themselves. But in these instances, I believe, we are seeing "taking" disguised as giving. These people allow others—people, careers, causes—to take from them. It has become a way of life, a behavioral pattern akin to reflexes, for them to sacrifice in this way. Giving of this type is often triggered or accompanied by feelings of sympathy for the other.

What is lacking in interactions of this sort is conscious awareness of motivation, reactions, sense of self, and personal limitations on the part of the giver. One can never truly give without this conscious awareness, and unless one can truly give, one can easily be taken from. Now let us turn our attention more specifically to the nature of giving in nursing.

Client Needfulness and Nurse Response

The situations and circumstances with which nurses must cope on a daily basis can certainly be difficult and taxing. We become witness to the tragedies of life and the delicacy of human existence. We are confronted with patients in pain, families in crisis, people needing so much that one wonders if they can ever be satisfied. In essence, whenever we are involved in nurse–client interactions, our clients want or need something that we have—our time, our compassion, our knowledge, our skill, our understanding. Remembering that the nurse is an energy field, we realize that all of these wants/needs are demands for our energy. How do nurses respond to this needfulness of clients? It seems that there are two primary modes of coping between which most nurses must choose in protecting their energies, the actual choice being made at a largely unconscious level. These two modes may be thought of as the *Defensive Mode* and the *Sympathetic Mode*. As it turns out, neither of these two modes is very effective in accomplishing the task at hand; namely, to protect the nurse from being drained through involvement with the client.

The Defensive Mode

When the demand for energy, the needfulness of the client, is received by the nurse-field, anxiety is aroused. To defend against being drained, the nurse utilizes a variety of defensive behaviors. These behaviors may include emotional distancing and withdrawal; avoidance of the client;

excessive task orientedness; derogatory labeling of clients as "demanding" or "uncooperative"; inappropriate levity and jocularity; false reassurance; or becoming angry with the client and thereby justifying avoidance. The possible behaviors that may be utilized as defense mechanisms are as varied as the nurses who use them.

In evaluating the effectiveness of this mode of coping, it is important to keep several points in mind:

1. We must remember that an energy field can never be completely closed off to the environment. Whether we are aware of it or not, we are continually exchanging energy with those around us. Thus, even when we are deliberately trying to cling to our own energies, energy may be taken from us.

2. Resisting interaction with the client is akin to the struggle over the apple discussed earlier. In trying to keep what is ours, in this case our energy, we are actually expending energy. It is a lot of work to maintain defense mechanisms, and a lot of energy is spent in attempting to do so.

3. Since this entire process is to varying degrees unconscious, it is beyond our conscious awareness, control, and regulation. We may end up feeling badly as a result of a struggle we didn't know we were involved in, and we will have no clue as to why we are feeling the way that we are.

4. This approach toward clients will most certainly conflict with what the nurse believes a nurse *should* be and do, and probably with his or her image of self as nurse. This conflict—again largely unconscious—saps more energy.

Thus, the end result for the nurse utilizing the Defensive Mode of coping with client needfulness is often fatique, guilt, and frustration, a kind of nurse burn-out (Fig. 14–1).

The Sympathetic Mode

In this mode, the reception of the signal of client needfulness triggers a reaction of sympathy in the nurse. Sympathy may be defined as "the quality of being affected by the state of another with feelings correspondent in kind." When the nurse feels sympathy for the client, there is an outpouring, a veritable flood of emotional energy given out to the client. The outward flow of energy is largely unregulated and uncontrolled, arising as it does from an intense, emotional need or desire to "make everything alright." Let us now consider the effect that this mode of coping has on the nurse.

Consider the implications of this mode of coping in terms of the definition of sympathy. In feeling sympathy, the nurse is literally

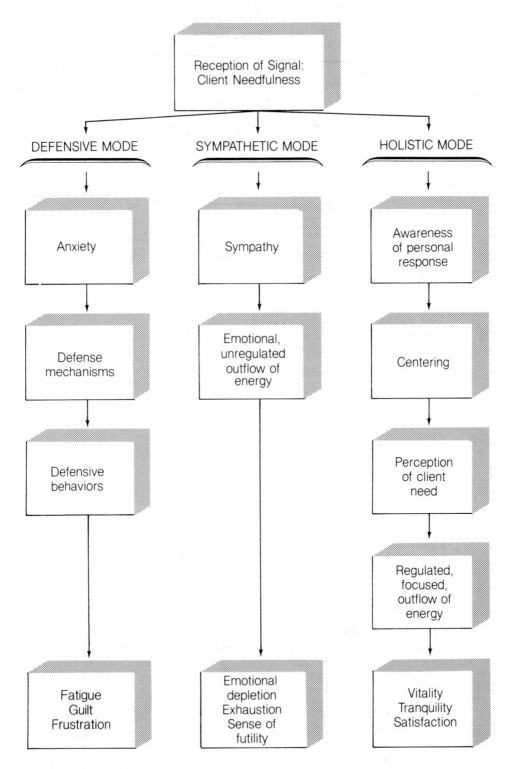

Figure 14-1.
Modes of coping.

allowing himself or herself to feel *as* the client does. The client's fears, pain, anxiety, depression, and so on become the nurse's. The transfer of these feelings occurs as the client-field and the nurse-field interact and penetrate each other, which they do continually. But in a sympathetic state, the nurse is taking in the emotionally charged energy of the client and retaining it, not dispersing it, or grounding it, if you will. The feelings of the client remain within the nurse, as so many of us realize when we return to our homes after working and can think only of this or that client in a sad and wrenching way.

In addition to taking in the "negative" energies of the client, the sympathetic response carries with it an outpouring of our own emotional energies. The combination of these two factors leaves the sympathetic nurse emotionally drained, exhausted, and, often, feeling futile, for in reality sympathy is of little use to even the client (Fig. 14–1).

This is the "emotional involvement" with clients about which we are so passionately warned by our teachers and our colleagues, and rightly so. It is not, however, the kind of involvement that has been discussed previously as part of a holistic approach to nursing intervention. It is this mode of coping, the Holistic Mode, that we will now explore.

The Holistic Mode

When a nurse is interacting from a holistic stance, he or she is interacting from a highly conscious and aware perspective. This awareness and sensitivity extend outwardly toward the client, as discussed above, but also penetrate inwardly toward the nurse-self. One cannot be more perceptive of the environment without also being more perceptive of self; conversely, one does not develop greater self-awareness without also becoming more sensitive to others in the process. As we shall see, it is this very phenomenon that serves to protect the nurse from being drained when interacting with clients in the Holistic Mode.

When the needfulness of the client is received through the nurse-client energy exchange, it is recognized at a conscious level because the nurse is in an open, perceptive state of awareness. By definition, the nurse in this state of awareness has access to his or her personal response to this message. This is a very significant advantage, for this awareness of a response can serve as a warning signal that there is potential for becoming drained at that moment. Thus, the nurse can take a few moments to regroup, to recenter, before proceeding any further with the client. In the centered state, the nurse's perceptivity to self and others is enhanced. It is as if the muting switch, referred to earlier, has been turned off. The vague awareness of the client's needfulness may become more defined so that a more precise understanding of the exact nature of the need is realized. Thus, centering serves a dual purpose: (1) to really focus in on the state of the client's energy field, and (2) to give the nurse conscious control of his or her energy exchange in response to the client's need.

In the centered state, the outflow of the nurse's energies becomes a conscious, focused, and regulated process, in contrast with the automatic, unconscious, and unregulated reactions that characterize the Defensive Mode and the Sympathetic Mode. (While our focus in this discussion is on the nurse, it should be pointed out that the client is certain to benefit more from a holistic interaction than from an interaction utilizing the Defensive Mode or Sympathetic Mode.)

In addition to the outward flow of energy, the nurse in an open, centered state of awareness is able to regulate the inward flow of energy from the environment in the following manner.

As has been discussed, an energy field is always exchanging energy with the environment. Whether or not we *perceive* that we are taking in energy from our environment, we are always *receiving* energy. However, this exchange or degree of openness to the environment may be influenced through the conscious awareness of the nurse. In an open, centered posture, the conscious nurse processes the signals that he or she receives, and so perception of the nature of these energies occurs. The perception of these energies is such that information about the client-field becomes evident. When the required information has been gathered, the nurse is able to release this energy, for it is no longer useful or helpful and in fact can be harmful, as we have discussed. In a centered and conscious state of awareness, the nurse can filter the energies and allow them to pass through him or her, in contrast to the unconscious retention of "negative" energies that can occur in the Defensive Mode or the Sympathetic Mode.

In addition, the centered nurse is able to consciously draw upon the vital energies in the environment that surrounds us, so that as he or she gives energy to the client, he or she is simultaneously replenished. Remember the anecdote about the apple: no one can take from you when you are truly giving.

Thus, in the Holistic Mode of coping with client needfulness, the nurse is able to regulate energy exchange with the client, such that the maximum therapeutic benefit is derived by the client, with simultaneous benefit for the nurse. Involvement with the client in the Holistic Mode usually results in feelings of vitality, tranquility, and satisfaction on the part of the nurse (Fig. 14–1).

Summary

Nursing within a holistic framework offers to us a unique opportunity and an exciting challenge.

The opportunity is to affect, to help our fellow man at the deepest levels of human existence. It provides us with the occasion to utilize our whole selves, with all of our knowledge, our creativity, and our caring in assisting people to grow toward higher levels of wellness. In using ourselves in this way and toward this end, we cannot help but to grow ourselves.

The challenge of holistic nursing must ultimately be one of expanding our self-knowledge. Involvement with people at the level that we have been discussing involves a commitment: a commitment to exploring our motivation for such involvement; a commitment to learning about our own limitations and frailties as human beings; a commitment to be honest with ourselves and to accept ourselves for who we really are without illusion; a commitment to explore our own depths so that we will not project our own fears and uncertainties onto our clients.

The process of knowing one's self may take a lifetime. We are never the same person for very long; we are always growing and changing. But the more deeply we come to know ourselves, the more deeply we can come to know, understand, and care for others. The beauty of nursing within a holistic framework is the realization that we are not really separate from our clients, that there is a mutuality in all of our interactions, through which we stand to gain every bit as much as the clients we nurse.

The challenge is enormous, but the satisfaction is immeasurable.

References

1. Rogers M: An Introduction to the Theoretical Basis of Nursing. Philadelphia, FA Davis, 1970
2. Yura H, Walsh M: The Nursing Process, 3rd ed. New York, Appleton-Century-Crofts, 1978
3. Krieger D: The Therapeutic Touch: How to Use Your Hands to Help or to Heal. Englewood Cliffs, Prentice-Hall, 1979

Suggested Readings

James M, Savary L: A New Self. Reading, Mass., Addison-Wesley, 1977
Jourard SM: The Transparent Self. New York, van Nostrand, 1971
Le Shan L: Alternate Realities, the Search for the Full Human Being. New York, Ballantine Books, 1976

Maslow AH: Toward a Psychology of Being. New York, van Nostrand, 1968

Maslow AH: The Farther Reaches of Human Nature. New York, Viking Press, 1971

May R: Man's Search for Himself. New York, Signet Books, 1953

Mayeroff M: On Caring. New York, Harper & Row, 1971

Rogers CR: On Becoming a Person. Boston, Haughton Mifflin, 1961

Stevens JO: Awareness: Exploring, Experimenting, Experiencing. New York, Bantam Books, 1971

15 We Are One: The Renaissance Nurse as Neighbor

Nancy E. Boyd

The basis of the concept of community described here is the belief stated in the previous chapters of this book: at the core of holistic health practices is a philosophy that *must be lived.* Renaissance Nursing is not a 40-hour-per-week job, but rather a 24-hour-a-day commitment. The Renaissance Nurse belongs to many "communities"—professional, spiritual, or residential, for example. This chapter will focus on nursing care provided to the neighborhood in which I have made my home for the past five years.

Significance for Nursing

Martha Rogers states that "the purpose of nursing is to help people achieve their maximum health potential. Nursing's first line of defense is promotion of health and prevention of illness. Care of the sick is resorted to when our first line of defense fails."[1] One of the most logical places to fulfill this purpose is in the neighborhood where one lives. Holistic health practices give the Renaissance Nurse the requisite tools to foster health and humaneness at the first line of defense. With the advent of a national health insurance program, the promotion of health at the community level may be viewed as less expensive and therefore more desirable than today's support of "illness care" by the medical–industrial complex.

Hodgman, in her 1970 study of nursing in a ghetto community action agency, noted that traditional approaches to health care related to urban poor and ghetto residents need rethinking because "there seems to be a discrepancy between what is known and what needs to be known" to best serve these populations.[2] The urban area considered in this chapter is underserved by the present health care delivery system and in this respect is representative of many similar communities.

My neighborhood is an ethnically and racially mixed community of persons of a broad range of ages, incomes, and religious and educational backgrounds. Among our predominantly black, Hispanic, and white population one finds persons who are unemployed, homemakers, blue-collar workers, owners of small businesses, white-collar workers, and professionals. Interracial couples, both heterosexual and homosexual, are respected neighbors, as is a lay religious community of gays which serves homosexual persons here and in other parts of the city. Conventional and storefront churches of Roman Catholic, Eastern Orthodox, and Pentecostal faiths, complemented by a Sikh ashram and Muslim mosques, are numerous.

We live in three- and four-story, nineteenth-century row houses and in city housing projects. Supermarkets are outside the immediate area, but small, family-owned grocery stores where Spanish-speaking residents can shop in their native tongue for ethnic foods dot almost every corner. Two public elementary schools are within an easy walk for neighborhood children. The senior-citizen center and daycare center bordering our area are used by few of our residents. The one city-run health center in our area is slated to be closed due to underutilization.

The social agencies that serve us are outside of the neighborhood, and they suffer the constraints of inefficient procedures, poorly trained personnel, and inadequate or misappropriated resources. Their representatives are often insensitive, disrespectful, or unresponsive to persons in need. Some ethnic- and religious-group members find that these Western-oriented social-welfare and health-care providers available to our community neither acknowledge nor honor their languages, belief systems, and special health needs. This lack of transcultural understanding is coupled with the experience that most agencies deal only with major problems and crises, not the day-to-day problems of how to cope. Emergency rooms and clinics of hospitals are used as the "family doctor" when an illness can no longer be managed at home.

Brisk illegal drug-retailing businesses involve many community residents as sellers, buyers, users, and robbery or burglary victims. The police department is understaffed and at times either powerless to effectively deal with the drug traffic or implicitly cooperative with organized crime. A variety of nearby detoxification programs is available to alcohol and controlled substance abusers, most involving a short hospital stay and outpatient follow-up. Although hospital emergency rooms and clinics do treat the illnesses and traumatic injuries of drug sellers and users, many persons are reluctant to seek this type of treatment for drug-related problems (even gunshot wounds!), fearing that they will be reported to law-enforcement agents.

Through interactions with neighbors, an inescapable awareness of my responsibility to implement nursing knowledges within my community grew. The need for direct intervention in the affairs of daily living and in the health care of those groups alienated by existing agencies became evident to me. The role of Renaissance Nurse as catalyst in two situations began to crystallize: (1) where individual community members assume responsibility for their own growth and health and (2) where the community as a whole deepens its meshwork of mutual understanding and respect, cooperation, and harmony among residents.

As Hodgman concluded, ". . . a lack of involvement, when involvement is necessary for the welfare of others to whom we feel a responsibility, can no longer be justified by excuses of professional detachment or research objectivity."[3] I hold myself accountable to my community and my peers for my actions and my failures to act.

Personal Philosophy

Meek, in *Healers and the Healing Process*, states as follows:

> We do not profess to understand at this time all of the precise mechanisms by which these emotions (empathy, harmony, unselfishness, devotion, tenderness, consecration, kindness, fellow-feeling, love and compassion) of the healer help the patient to re-energize the weakened or diseased cells of his body but there can be no longer any doubt that love and compassion are the cornerstones of the edifice of health, healing, and wholeness.[4]

In a similar vein, LeShan firmly and provocatively ends *The Medium, the Mystic, and the Physicist* with the following statement:

> It seems to me that the challenge to science, to man, to the human experiment is, finally and irrevocably, whether or not man can accept that he is a part of the energy of the universe and can only function harmoniously within it through his capacity to love—infinitely.[5]

All participation in community health care described here was voluntary and integrated with the participants' own personal lives and work. Any increasing perception of the needs of others or growing ability to affect change has been concurrent with a daily dedication to creating in the environment an atmosphere of serene, accepting love. I personally consider that attempts to do this must have priority over excellence at work, success in relationships, and recognition for achievements. This conviction arises out of a belief that, in terms of universal laws, love is a basic, underlying force which creates wholeness, harmony, and order within and among living beings, and, as such, takes precedence over personal goals.

This love makes real a condition of existence where all living

beings are equal. No being is better than or less worthwhile than
another. Each individual incorporates all aspects of being, crowding the
entire spectrum of human values from "excellent" and "best" to "evil"
and "bad." Each person, animal, insect, plant, and microbe is regarded
as having within itself a center of life which reflects the power, order,
and harmonious design of the universe. Thus, we can only acknowledge
that we are one with every other living being, and they one with us, in
this condition of love. Recognition of an individual's dignity, worth,
and fellowship is automatically accorded the drug-pusher, the elderly
widow, the concerned homeowner, and the starving stray dog alike.

Conflicts of interest between living beings are omnipresent
manifestations of the complexity and diversity of existence (*e.g.,*
between humans and the animals or plants to be killed for their food,
or between a neonate and the bacteria proliferating in the neonate's
cerebrospinal fluid). A universal response is to "choose sides"—to
consider the more evolved living being "right" or more valued and the
less evolved being "wrong" or less valued. Renaissance Nurses find
themselves in the awesome position of supporting all forms of life with
deference and love, while realizing that the life process in humans
dictates actions that affect the quality and quantity of life of other
living beings.

Theoretical Framework

Assumptions from nursing's conceptual model developed by Martha
Rogers (see Chap. 8) provide the most appropriate frame of reference
from which the Renaissance Nurse may derive holistic health practices.
The human is held to be a unified whole, different from and greater
than the sum of his parts. The fundamental unit of the living system is
an energy field having a nonapparent "fourth" dimension. The human
field interacts as a whole with the environment, which is also an
energy field. Continuous change typifies the mutual, simultaneous
interactions between the human energy field and the environmental
energy field. Energy fields are identified by their pattern and
organization. The character of the complementary changes human and
environmental fields undergo is associated with the pattern and
organization of the fields as well as with other variables, including field
boundaries, structure, function, rhythmicity, energy exchanges, and
position in space–time.[6]

An analysis of holistic health methods used in our multifaceted
community situation reveals three types of healing: (1) Therapeutic
Touch, which was used mostly to treat physical problems, (2) a non-
touch metaphysical interaction used to stimulate personal evolution and

transformation, and (3) another metaphysical interaction in which the all-consuming oneness of the universe is effected. Those of us consciously working together to create health and wholeness in our neighborhood have been excited by the individual growth and community progress toward understanding and cooperation we have seen. We believe that our neighborhood is a model for the more harmonious way in which humans and environment can function as worldwide communication brings people closer together and as global problems intensify.

The discussion of healing must be initiated by first mentioning misunderstandings that may be generated by the terms *healer* and *healee*. The former designates a person who brings therapeutic interventions, in this case certain holistic health practices, to bear in a situation where evaluation of data has led to an assessment indicating that the interventions would be appropriate. The latter identifies the living being or community of living beings toward whom these interventions are directed and with whom the healer enters into a mutual, simultaneous interaction. However, as with any other therapy, the practitioner can only offer or extend healing as a tool to clients, who may be able to use this support in their own dynamic processes to achieve further growth and a more efficient state of well-being.

What subsequently occurs will be determined by the algebraic summation of the pluses and minuses of all possibilities existing for the client at that point in his interaction with the environment. The practitioner does not "heal" anyone; clients heal themselves, perhaps using the supports extended.

With this clarified, Yogi Ramacharaka's comments in *Psychic Healing* provide the setting:

> Have confidence in yourself, and in your healing power. It is . . . not a gift bestowed upon but a few. It is a general gift and natural power that may be developed by practice and confidence, and instead of decreasing by use, it grows in proportion to its use. It is like a muscle that is developed by practice. . . .[7]

Dora Kunz gives three prerequisites for acting as a healer, which echo Meek's beliefs: (1) have compassion for the healee, (2) believe that you are effective in helping the healee, and (3) leave your ego and personal interests out of the healing interaction.[8] In all healing interactions, the response of the healee is dependent upon whether or not "the patient will change his or her habits of living, and will endeavor to live in accordance with Nature's laws," not upon the effectiveness of the healer alone.[9] Development of habits of daily meditation, prayer, or contemplation of universal power and order by the healer is usually concomitant with an interest in using holistic health practices.

The Medical Group of the Theosophical Research Centre in London defines health and healing as follows:

> *Normal health may be said to be present when a person is at peace with himself and is in a harmonious relationship with his whole environment. . . .* From this it naturally follows that the process of healing, whatever may be the particular method employed or the field of activity involved, should be regarded fundamentally as the restoration of the normal relationships already mentioned.[10]

Everywhere in our environment we see evidences of ordering and patterning forces manifest in matter: the vibrations of atoms, space lattices, sea shells, human biorhythms, the whirl of galaxies. While using the first healing method, Therapeutic Touch, I think of channeling the capacity of these natural ordering and harmonizing influences, which affect matter or systems, to the living energy field (human, animal, plant, *etc.*) that is in a state of relative disharmony. These natural influences with ability to order may themselves be field phenomena. In interaction with a subject's energy field, their capacity to do work will be called *energy.*

Dolores Krieger describes the act of healing as follows:

> . . . The channeling of this energy flow by the healer for the supplementation of that of the ill individual. On the physical level I felt that this occurs by electron transfer resonance. The resonance would act in the service of the ill person to reestablish the vitality of the flow in this open system, to restore, as it were, unimpeded communication with the environment—for given this, all literature agrees, the patient really heals himself.[11]

The healing method used most commonly to assess and treat physical and emotional complaints is similar to Krieger's Therapeutic Touch,[12] pranic healing described by Ramacharaka,[13] the laying on of hands or vital magnetic treament described by the Medical Group,[14] and a combination of Meek's Type "A" and Type "B" healing.[15]

This healing method resembles that which LeShan calls Type 2 healing, where:

> [The healer] perceives a pattern of activity between his palms when his hands are "turned on" and facing each other. Some healers perceive this as a "flow of energy," some as a sphere of activity. The hands are so placed—one on each side of the healee's pathological area—so that this "flow of energy" is perceived to "pass through" the troubled area. This is usually conceived of by the healer as "healing energy" which "cures" or "treats" the sick area. . . . In Type 2 the healer *tries* to heal; he wants to and attempts to do so through the "healing flow."[16]

There are times and circumstances, however, when it is not appropriate to touch or hold one's hands near the client. Problems clients face in attempting to change their life-styles, their ways of coping and of attaining gratification, and the ways in which they view themselves exist more in the emotional, mental, and spiritual realms of being, with reflections in the physical. The method employed in such instances is similar to Ramacharaka's metaphysical healing,[17] the Medical Group's mental healing,[18] and Meek's Type "C."[19] LeShan also identifies a healing method, called Type 1, where "the healer goes into an altered state of consciousness in which he views himself and the healee as one entity."[20] He states as follows:

> What appeared to happen in Type 1 healing was that because he was momentarily in an "ideal organismic situation," the healee's self-repair and self-recuperative systems began to operate at a level closer than usual to their potential. Type 1 psychic healing was not a "doing something" to the healee, but a meeting and uniting with him on a profound level, a uniting that permitted something new to happen. . . .[21]

In this union, where both healer and healee are whole, the full integration of a person's higher spiritual self with his or her existence in this time and place is fact. This type of healing can be readily employed with persons with whom one may not have direct contact (e.g., those neighbors one may not know personally, the members of organized crime, and plain-clothes detectives).

LeShan goes on to say that "the uniting leads to ESP-types of perceptions, and since there is no bar to the flow of information within the one entity that now exists, these perceptions are often remembered on return to the Sensory Reality."[22] Among fellow nurse–healers and myself, we find that subjective impressions of the healee's energy field come into our awareness with increasing frequency. These impressions take many forms, such as visualizations, or a knowledge of the healee's personal background, interpersonal relationships, or emotional hang-ups which have not been otherwise communicated. To date, no substantive and controlled research has been done on these subjective visualizations, and so they are offered for what they are: personal impressions.

Another type of healing has been noted by LeShan which "calls for a type of change *beyond* the body's ability at self-repair."[23] He describes this Type 5 healing as where:

> . . . The healer knows that he is a part of the whole cosmos as a wave is part of the ocean. There is no separation between him and the rest of the universe, yet he is a unique part. The All affects him as he affects the All. The healee is also part of the All in the

same way. The healee is, so to speak, another wave. In this state of consciousness, the healer knows that he is distinct from the healee although both are a part of the same ocean and thereby connected. In moments of the pure knowledge of this, the healer mentally attempts to bring the immense resources of the harmonic energies of the cosmos to bear on the healee, and thus to increase his inner and outer harmony.[24]

Ramacharaka also speaks about "a highest form of healing," where cures "are often practically *instantaneous*, although it does not necessarily follow that they must be so."[25]

Ramacharaka cautions that this kind of healing "is much rarer and less common than is generally believed to be the case."[26] LeShan confesses to "feeling remarkably tentative" as he writes about the Transpsychic Reality in which Type 5 healing occurs.[27] However, the benefits of such a method to living beings—individually and in communion with one another—are obvious. One might possibly tap it in situations where one is using Type 1 healing. Ramacharaka says:

> Do not be afraid to try this form of treatment—provided you do it in the right spirit. And you will find that you will become a greater and greater instrument for the expression of [it] as time goes on. . . .[28]

He also states that it "cannot be mis-applied or prostituted in cases of relief to suffering humanity . . ."[29]

LeShan reassures us:

> . . . I do not believe it is possible to use these energies to harm. You can only get in touch with them when you are willing to give up your usual sense of identity, when you want to be *more* in harmony with the rest of the universe rather than less in harmony. . . . To "hurt" or to "harm" is to reduce harmony, not add to it. To "heal" is to increase inner and outer harmony, not lessen it.[30]

Armed with this encouragement, I value and attempt to realize this form of healing more and more as a responsible resident of our planet.

The distinctions drawn between various healing methods in efforts to establish a theoretical rationale for healing may not hold in actual practice. Every Renaissance Nurse has a unique understanding of and approach to healing, as is evident in other chapters of this book. An overlapping of methods is inevitable as each nurse employs holistic health practices in the care of individuals, families, communities, and other living beings. The Renaissance Nurse's perceptions and skill in the art of healing continuously evolve in pace with increasing personal insight and wholeness. Therapeutic Touch, as it is being developed by

Krieger, encompasses some of LeShan's Type 1 and Type 5 techniques, in addition to being frankly similar to Type 2 healing, I believe.

Practical Application

My involvement with and commitment to my community's well-being began three years ago. Isaac M., a 26-year-old Puerto Rican male with a 9-year history of drug abuse, ran a "shooting gallery" in the furnished room of a row house on the same block where I live. To support a habit or heroin and cocaine abuse, Isaac sold heroin, cocaine, and other controlled substances, and then let buyers use the privacy of his room to self-administer the drugs, or "shoot up."

Juan M. was shot in the back in the middle of our block by an acquaintance to whom he was indebted over narcotics and who had been stabbed by Juan's brother in a fight. A month later, Willie, the owner of the corner bodega, was shot and killed during a robbery of his grocery store. Believing that Isaac's drug dealings on our block would lead only to more violence and would create an unsafe atmosphere in which to live and raise children, block association members decided to take action.

They explained their fears to Isaac and asked him to either clean up his activities or move. They also made a spontaneous offer to help him if he wanted to get off drugs. Anxious to prod Isaac into action, they explained that the block association would picket in front of his house the following week if he did not comply. During the intervening week, it was business as usual in Isaac's rented room. The picketers, representative of the white, black, and Hispanic population of our block, soon turned away one of Isaac's prospective customers, and Isaac had to hurry down the block in the direction in which his sale had disappeared.

The next week, dissatisfied with Isaac's lack of cooperation and knowing he owed his landlady eight weeks rent, a lawyer on the block instituted eviction proceedings against Isaac. When the city marshal arrived to dispossess him, it was learned that Isaac, to everyone's surprise, had signed himself into the detoxification center of a city hospital. We subsequently learned that addicts often seek treatment voluntarily when they are facing imminent arrest or other social and legal pressures.

Three neighbors had decided among themselves to offer Isaac an alternative life-style after his discharge the next week, when he would find himself without a place to live and without belongings. Of this group of three, two had had drug dependencies. They outlined a program they had been talking about for months and now saw as coming alive to assist Isaac in his hour of emptiness. Upon completion of detoxification, the ex-addict would sit down with the group and together they would draw up a program to meet his spiritual, emotional, physical, educational, economic, social, and legal needs. Psychotherapy and school would be required components. The group would make referrals to appropriate existing professional agencies; act as advocates for the ex-addict; and offer love, support, and companionship to him in the neighborhood where he lives. Ex-addicts could stay in the mainstream of community life while being assisted to adopt an alternative way of living.

The three wanted to know if I would be interested in helping them, starting the next day when Isaac would be discharged. I had never before seriously considered living my belief that we are all one in the street with drug traffickers! A friend once said that the more you know, the less choice you have. There was no choice. I began to live my "we are one" words in a new dimension. I will always be grateful to the three outstanding people who brought me this opportunity.

Excerpts from a poem and photographic essay called, appropriately, *Please Touch,* by McMahon and Campbell, capture that moment:

> We think of religious activity directed toward God
>   —instead of man.
> We believe in someone divine rather than in ourselves.
> Maybe we have turned religion inside out . . .
> Can we turn "touching" inside-out to find man—and God? . . .
> People really want to believe in themselves and one another . . .
> We do not come to believe in ourselves until someone reveals
>   that deep inside us something is valuable—worth listening
>   to—worthy of our trust—sacred to our touch.
> And yet, isolation and loneliness, greed, suspicion, hate
>   are experiences around us—and within us—evil everywhere
>   mingled with the beautiful. . . .
> The needs of others call us to be life-source—find light in
>   the dark—in sparks of human goodness alive beneath
>   encrusted surfaces.
> Can we so communicate belief in the basic goodness of people
>   that they come to believe in themselves?—mutually discovering
>   that "the light shines on in the dark and the darkness has
>   never quenched it." (John 1:5)
> We must learn to celebrate life where we find it.
> We are all a community presence—an extension of the loving
>   community or the rejecting closed community that has made
>   us what we are. . . .
> Love is the extension of God's community into the world,
>   into us. . . .

> Revelation appears from within—the experience of ourselves
> as a community expression that is human—and divine. . . .
> Fascination, creativity, going one step beyond, succeeding
> where all odds are against us, probing for answers to all
> the questions life puts to us.
> Men will recognize that they are most deeply involved with
> God when they touch the world around them as invitation—
> and respond with a confident "Amen."[31]

Isaac's most immediate needs were for a place to live, people to believe in him, financial assistance, and someone to go with him as he faced an indictment for stealing a tape deck from a parked van. Without the explicit knowledge that Isaac had made three previous attempts to stay drug-free since he started taking drugs at the age of 17, we were well aware of the decidedly discouraging probability that Isaac would not stay out of trouble.

We acknowledged to ourselves the risks to which we would expose our persons and property in opening our lives and giving of our love in a street setting that lacks the safeguards of office walls and undisclosed private lives. We also shared a deep commitment to the concept that we are all one; that people do need someone to believe in them when they feel their situation is hopeless and their problems overwhelming; that people have to be touched and hugged; and that love is the only thing that "will get you over." We chose to offer ourselves, our support, and our service to Isaac, realizing that without help Isaac's chances of making it by himself were even slimmer than with our help.

Upon his release from the hospital, a group member took Isaac into her home pending his finding an apartment of his own. A list of goals, problems to be solved, and scheduled activities was drawn up with Isaac. Daily contact with core group members for counselling, dealing with issues as they arose, therapeutic interventions and healing, and evaluation was on a scheduled and an as-neeeded basis. In the early weeks we found ourselves putting in 20-hour days. Hodgman, too, found that "it appeared as if my time and energy were almost totally spent in coping with the very practical problems that consistently arose and had to be dealt with."[32]

Block residents generously volunteered time, help, and goods to Isaac. His original activities included tutoring by an elementary school teacher, yoga lessons (to which he was given a free scholarship by the people who owned the van he vandalized), being catcher on a baseball team that met weekly, a bilingual college-preparatory course at the YMCA, and weekly art lessons. These activities were designed by Isaac to build on his years of semiprofessional baseball in Puerto Rico and his one year of college-level education in architecture. Through Aspira, an organization that promotes higher education for persons of Hispanic origin, Isaac made plans to enter a bilingual program in radiographic technology offered by a city college when he finished the YMCA's course.

Responding to community backing of Isaac, a landlord rented him a one-bedroom apartment across the street from me. Furniture, dishes, paintings, plants, and elbow grease were donated in an outpouring of community spirit. Three Puerto Rican families on the block issued Isaac invitations to dinner on a regular basis. As long as he desired it, someone accompanied Isaac to welfare, court, probation, and therapy appointments as friend and advocate.

Isaac, as well as those who later joined our program, had many physical and emotional complaints. These were more pronounced in the period immediately after detoxification. Chief among the complaints were feelings of nervousness, insomnia, nasal congestion, stomach pains, and pain in an old gunshot wound site. To promote relaxation, facilitate gastrointestinal function, relieve pain, and so on, the first healing method, resembling closely Therapeutic Touch and LeShan's Type 2 healing, was employed. Isaac found these measures were effective in relieving pain and in promoting relaxation and sleep. A fellow ex-addict explained that he found nothing unusual in the motions used in Therapeutic Touch because his Puerto Rican grandmother used a similar form of healing.

The very rich, intense experience of sharing Isaac's life so intimately during his period of transition did not occur in a vacuum. Despite our preoccupations with Isaac's hour-by-hour existence, we soon were forcefully reminded that all of this was ocurring in the fabric of the community in which we lived. Block association meetings became a forum where people dismayed to find Isaac was still on our block could express their fears. ("What if he goes back to drugs and starts robbing again? I have a 100-thousand dollar house and he's living next door!") Drug sellers on the corner were sure that when they were hassled by the police it was a result of information we passed along from Isaac to the precinct. Although remaining neutral in their stance, we knew organized crime members were completely informed about our activities with Isaac.

The local police, widely known to have a comfortable, working relationship with both the street drug people and organized crime, facilitated by a corrupt precinct captain, began to make us feel we were living a grade-B version of *Serpico*. Anxious that we not upset the *status quo*, plain-clothes detectives began to watch our houses. They wanted to know if we were going to become involved in selling drugs and if we had plans to reveal any information we had learned to the public. They added levity to the situation. Have you ever seen grown men sitting on the steps of a brownstone house holding paper bags with two-way radio antennae sticking out of the top and raising these bags to their ears?

Outside of television viewing, our inexperience with these activities predisposed us to some nervousness and diarrhea initially. As it became clear that our surveillance, which almost certainly included tapping of our telephones, was not leading to other forms of harassment, we relaxed.

LeShan's Type 1 (and possibly Type 5) healing was appropriately directed toward concerned neighbors, street-corner drug pushers, members of organized crime, and police officers. A retrospective of day-to-day victories and setbacks reveals an overall trend toward constructive interactions. The detectives began to chat with us and even sought our help in finding homes for the sergeant's kittens. We hailed their familiar, beat-up car for their assistance when a lost 4-year-old child appeared on our steps. Our precinct got a new captain. Many drug pushers of long-standing were put in prison. Another was considering giving up "the business." The swirls of new faces to replace the old came and went with a rapidity that robbed the illegal drug industry of the stability it once had in our neighborhood.

As word of our endeavors spread, neighbors from several walks of life, with a wide variety of problems and requests, began to approach us. It soon became apparent that our project, which we called "We Are One," would not be confined to serving ex-addicts. It would have a changing character as our actions continued to be geared to meet our two umbrella objectives:

1. To assist clients to assume responsibility for achieving optimal self-actualization

2. To strengthen within our community constructive and cooperative interactions among residents, based on mutual understanding and respect

After six months of staying "clean," Isaac slipped into heroin abuse again, supporting his habit by pushing drugs. We had long before realized that our emotional responses to Isaac's successes and failures had to be recognized and, then, divested of our personal attachment, be allowed to dissipate.

TO ISAAC:

You are very young
and very old
and sweet
and full of bullshit.

You spot pins in shag carpet,
money dropped a pew away in church,
and open car doors,
but you don't see the buds on trees.

How can someone who has
held a gun to people's temples
look so guilty when telling a lie?

You ran a shooting gallery
yet three hours of school a day
and paying bills
are too complicated.

You angrily insist on doing what you want
but you'd rather cop out than tell someone no.

Didn't you know cold, sweaty fear
when you were shot?
Where is it hidden when you're tenderly
pushing Chino's little girl on the swing?

You're in trouble in the street—
you still owe Raoul a gun—
but it's the metaphysical awareness
welling up inside you in yoga class
that you run away from.

Was that the real you
painstakingly composting the garden,
chopping trees side by side with Boris,
sharing open love beyond that
which any single person can give?

We love you!

How can we help you?

In the use of any holistic healing method, it must be offered with compassion and skill, but without concern for the results. We committed ourselves to the principle that love, support, and assistance are the rights of all living beings, regardless of value judgments assigned to their behaviors.

Isaac continued to seek us out almost daily. He seemed grateful for our continuing acceptance of him even as we reflected his behavior for him to see and held up alternatives. Isaac made the decision to go to Puerto Rico with the young woman he loved and lived with, knowing that drug abusers face severe treatment on the island. He again got off of drugs and held a job as a construction worker. It was in his mother's village, more than two and a half years after our initial contact with Isaac, that he was shot in the back and killed by a man he had double-crossed when both were teenagers.

Guidelines for Holistic Community Health

The holistic process of growth that has occurred in our community can be integrated with guidelines for cross-cultural health programs developed by Project HOPE.[33] These guidelines have been adapted and are discussed here because of their value to the Renaissance Nurse who accepts responsibility for a loving, caring role in our shrinking world.

   1. *Be aware of the temptation to arrive with a specific plan of intervention.*

Intervention should be related to needs perceived by community members rather than planned by health professionals "who know best" what is "good" for the neighborhood. Recognize that other groups may have value systems different from your own; respect the differences. Our group's preconceived plan for helping ex-addicts to repattern their life-styles underwent its first revision when we sat down with Isaac to explore his problems and desires.

The importance of this approach was emphasized when Chino, a drug seller and user, angrily said he would have nothing to do with us because we were trying to "make Isaac white." After Isaac described his individually tailored program and it became evident that We Are One's objective was to help Isaac achieve his stated goals within the Puerto Rican–New Yorker culture, Chino began to ask us for instructions in the care of his 2½-year-old daughter.

   2. *Develop an awareness of your own culture and values.*

You must be accepted as a person before you will be accepted as a professional with services to offer. The first step is to critically and honestly appraise your own prejudices and value system. Do we see ourselves as better than or superior to the drug pusher or welfare mother? Can we lay aside our hierarchies of worth and allow the reality that we are truly one with our clients to flourish within our hearts as well as our minds?

As Hodgman also discovered, we found that our personal safety was assured once our credibility was established. Clients from a different culture will be acutely sensitive to the degree of consistency and straightforwardness with which you present yourself. Once Chino felt we were being open and up-front with everyone, he made a point of telling us that "you have nothing to worry about," meaning that word had been passed in the street that we were not to be harmed.

   3. *Familiarize yourself with the community.*

Where are the boundaries? What is the structure of the community (*e.g.*, buildings, stores, schools, fire houses, streets, subways)? How does the community function (*e.g.*, employment, transportation, families, public services)? What is the community's pattern (*e.g.*, cultural and ethnic groups, age distribution)? How is the community organized (*e.g.*, planning boards, associations, social clubs, retail businesses, residential interests)?

What are the sources of energy into the community (*e.g.*, religious and charitable organizations, food and fuel supplies, funding, stores)? Where is energy expended (*e.g.*, maintenance, education, production, discord and dissatisfactions)? What are the community's rhythms (*e.g.*, hours of work and business, day and night activities, seasonal changes)? Evaluate the integrity of human and environment energy fields (*e.g.*, dependability, consistency, maturity, interrelationships).

Our neighborhood pulses as children throng to and from school, adults surge to and from work, and social clubs light up and tune up in the evening. The social club is closing at 4 A.M. when the ashram begins its day with prayer and yoga. Summertime promotes social interactions on stoops and sidewalks; cold weather drives people into family homes, clubs, and the bodegas. Ethnic groups have permeable boundaries, accepting information about life-styles different from their own.

4. *Identify your own competencies and areas of deficiency.*

Another critical appraisal, this time of your professional assets and weaknesses, will guide you in making realistic commitments. Make the delimitations of your role clear. Anticipate areas in which conflicts of interest could develop (*e.g.*, in loaning of money, in the establishment of close personal relationships). Once the boundaries of your professional competence have been defined, effective referral of the client to the appropriate resource can take place. The Renaissance Nurse cannot overlook his or her responsibility to use holistic health methods knowledgeably and intelligently.

5. *Identify resources within the community.*

What services are available? What areas of expertise do community residents have? We Are One found that mutual cooperation on a variety of problems with St. Matthew's (the religious community serving gays), the Sikh ashram, the Spanish-language Roman Catholic chapel, and the Suni Moslem mosque, for example, had a synergistic effect in reaching satisfactory solutions. Botanicas, Aspira, relatives, and interested professionals all proved of invaluable assistance in various situations. A Young Puerto Rican couple who had just had their first baby, responded favorably to a suggestion that they check in on an elderly, Spanish-speaking widow who lived alone and was in failing health.

6. *Identify what you have to offer.*

When the community is aware of what you can do for them, what your overall objectives are, and what the delimitations of your service are, members will be able to make an informed choice about whether or not you would be able to help them with their aspirations, dreams, and difficulties.

We Are One came into being when group members established an accepting, approachable, respecting, loving, and helping *presence* in the streets and homes of our neighborhood in response to a perceived need. The services we offer fall into four main categories: (1) personal counseling; (2) health care and education; (3) matching needs to appropriate resources and sending available assistance to places where it is needed; and (4) improving communication and understanding through interpretation of behaviors, mores, and perspectives.

We have counseled persons with problems running the gamut from a child habitually late for school to a case of blackmail. Healing interventions and health education have been applied to numerous situations, from requests for contraception information to care of gunshot wounds. Connections between providers and consumers of various services facilitated by We Are One include the distribution of second-hand clothing and furniture scavenged from neighborhood waste cans. We function, when necessary, as advocate and friend to clients referred to other agencies.

The following vignette illustrates the role of interpretation and communication in community affairs. A white, middle-class neighbor discovered a drunken Hispanic man banging with fists on his car. The owner loudly demanded in English that the man, who was yelling in Spanish, stop assaulting his car. When the man resumed the activity a short while later, the owner came out of his house with a baseball bat. He was accompanied this time by his wife, who had a camera to record the man hitting the car. The drunken man pulled out a knife. The car owner, taking this gesture as an attack, began to hit the man with the bat. The man slashed the car owner's arm with his knife. The car owner was not aware that possession and display of a knife or gun are an important expression of manhood in many Hispanic cultures and not necessarily an indication that the weapon carrier has intentions of attacking. The car owner had misread the cues and instead wound up initiating the attack himself. A discussion of the events between the car owner and members of the social club, in front of which the car was parked, brought out the miscommunication. Neither party pressed charges.

7. Be flexible and compromise.

Any program offering services to the community must be dynamic and responsive to residents. Be aware that personal and emotional investment in either the process or its outcomes may prohibit you from recognizing changing needs and from letting go of functions that are no longer necessary.

As the roles that We Are One fulfilled continued to vary with the self-determined requests of community members, our acceptance within the community grew. Within a year's time, one staunch opponent of the group's support of addicts and ex-addicts turned over his house keys to a group member who agreed to walk his dog while the family was away. Another antagonist asked for evaluation of a painful ankle. Both men had snubbed group members in early months of We Are One, refusing even to say hello in the street. It is difficult to determine what role LeShan's Type 1 healing played in these attitudinal changes.

We Are One has undergone a further metamorphosis. It has merged membership and functions with the Universal Growth Center, which was recently started by a man who has given over life and house to community service.

8. *Work with circumstances as they exist.*

Accept the values and positions of community members. Rather than trying to change attitudes and behaviors, plan interventions within the present situation. If we had demanded that Isaac remain drug-free, we would have lost our opportunity for continued therapeutic intervention. Equipment, facilities, and personnel are often not what textbook authors envision; improvise with what is at hand. Calling on persons without education or experience to work with you under supervision may open new horizons for them in terms of capabilities, self-image, and even vocation.

9. *Timing is important.*

Constant assessment of current community patterns and evaluation of the appropriateness and effectiveness of measures implemented are crucial to successful attainment of your objectives. Capitalize on neighborhood rhythms and energy inputs when timing intervention. The Renaissance Nurse can expand traditional criteria for evaluation to include the subjective impressions accompanying LeShan's Type 1 healing.

A rule of thumb for evaluating the appropriateness of one's actions is to look at the fruits your efforts bear. If you constantly meet with friction, obstacles, and failure, it is time to reexamine your expectations and critically inspect your procedure from beginning to end.

10. *Set short-term goals within a framework of long-term goals.*

Failure to deal with the day-to-day problems of community members may discourage the community from choosing the services you offer. Meeting the short-term needs of a community gives you the opportunity to work on long-term goals and provides a period of exposure during which you can facilitate the integration of the neighborhood's potential for harmony and productive interaction through holistic health practices, such as LeShan's Type 1 and Type 5 healing methods.

The Renaissance Nurse, acting alone or in concert with others, can enhance the health, harmony, and productivity of any community once he or she becomes aware that each one of us is life-brother to all living beings and that we are each our brother's keeper.

References

1. Rogers ME: A symposium: approaches to doctoral preparation for nurses. Doctoral education in nursing. Nursing Forum 5:76
2. Hodgman: Nursing in a Community Action Agency—an Experience With Ghetto Teenagers, p. 22. New York, National League for Nursing, Department of Public Health Nursing, 1970
3. Hodgman, *ibid*, p 76
4. Meek GW: Toward a general theory of healing. In Meek GW (ed): *Healers and the Healing Process*, Wheaton, Ill.,: The Theosophical Publishing House, 1977, 231
5. LeShan L: The Medium, the Mystic and the Physicist: Towards a General Theory of the Paranormal. New York, Viking; 1974
6. Rogers ME: An Introduction to the Theoretical Basis of Nursing, p 92. Philadelphia, FA Davis, 1970
7. Yogi Ramacharaka: The Science of Psychic Healing, pp 13–14. Chicago, Yogi Publication Society, 1937
8. Kunz D: Healers' Workshop, Pumpkin Hollow Farm, Craryville, New York, August, 1974
9. Ramacharaka, *op cit*, p 12
10. The Medical Group, Theosophical Research Centre: The Mystery of Healing, p 6. Wheaton, Ill, the Theosophical Publishing House, 1958
11. Krieger D: Therapeutic Touch: a mode of primary healing based on a holistic concern for man. In The Physician of the Future Conference, International Cooperation Council, p 5. San Diego, California, June 21, 1975
12. Krieger, *op cit*
13. Ramacharaka, *op cit*, p 52
14. The Medical Group, *op cit*, pp 52–56
15. Meek, *op cit*, pp 214–221
16. LeShan, *op cit*, pp 112–113
17. Ramacharaka, *op cit*, pp 171–172
18. The Medical Group, *op cit*, p 56
19. Meek, *op cit*, pp 221–226
20. LeShan, *op cit*, p 106
21. LeShan, *op cit*, pp 110–111
22. LeShan, *op cit*, p 160
23. LeShan, *op cit*, p 156
24. LeShan, *op cit*, p 148
25. Ramacharaka, *op cit*, pp 174–175
26. Ramacharaka, *op cit*, p 174

27. LeShan, *op cit*, p 161
28. Ramacharaka, *op cit*, pp 183–184
29. Ramacharaka, *op cit*, p 178
30. LeShan, *op cit*, pp 162–163
31. McMahon EM, Campbell PA: Please Touch. United States of America, a Search Book by Sheed and Ward, 1969
32. Hodgman, *op cit*, p 22
33. Aeschliman D: Guidelines for cross-cultural health programs. Nursing Outlook 21:660, 1973

16 Holistic Health for the Elders

Catherine Salveson

Nursing and Aging in America Today

In our complex, secularized, fast-paced society, there are few things everyone has in common. One thing we all share is aging. No matter who you are, how much wealth, education or power you possess, each day you grow older and one day you will count yourself among the elderly. We can also look forward to an increasingly larger number of older people among us. In 1900 there were slightly more than 3 million elderly persons. By 1979 there were over 20 million. Projections indicate that 20% of the population will be 65 and over by the year 2000.[1]

The true facts about the elderly belie the social attitude of "failing" into old age. Ninety-five percent of people over 65 live successfully in the community—in rural areas or central cities. Only 5% are institutionalized. The number and proportion of the aged are new and fast-growing phenomena in our society. Between 1960 and 1974, the number of people aged 65 to 74 increased 23%; the number over 75 increased 49%. This is in contrast to an 11.5% increase in people under 45. Today, every tenth American is over 65.[2] Couple these statistics with the reality that older people often have multiple, chronic health problems, and we can begin to understand the growing concern among health planners for how these people will be taken care of. The way is open for new ways of caring. These include ancient as well as newly conceived methods that do not require expensive technologically based medicine but are based on the inherent natural power of the body to balance itself.

The prevalent attitude in medical care is to look back in the other direction and focus on the young. "Why treat someone who is 86 years old, he'll probably die soon anyway." Nursing the elderly has been viewed in the past as "second-class nursing," clearly not as important or prestigious as medical-surgical, intensive care unit, or coronary care unit work. It has only been since the implementation of Medicare and Medicaid that the profession of geriatric nursing has been recognized as

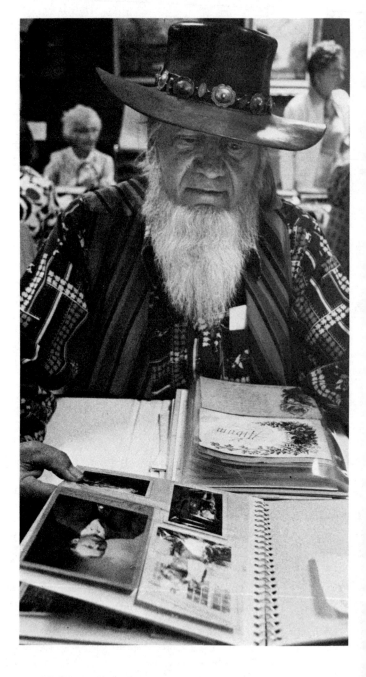

Fig. 16-1.
Older people like to
reminisce. In some of their
groups they can do this by
sharing photograph albums.
(Photo by Joe Dimas)

a clinical nursing specialty as well as a community and home care
practice. In 1971 there were over 40,000 registered nurses employed
full-time in nursing homes.[3] This figure does not include the home care
and public health nurses who minister to the 95% of the elderly who

still live at home. As more nurses become involved in the care of the aging among us, it is important to understand a change that is occurring in our attitudes toward our elders.

Our attitudes about nursing and caring for older people are merely an extension of our general feelings about aging. Growing older is seen by some as a disease in itself, something to fight against and overcome. Aging is used to explain disease and disease to explain aging.

Alex Comfort shares with us the stereotype of the ideal aged American as past folklore present it:

> He or she is a white-haired, inactive, unemployed person, making no demands on anyone, least of all the family, docile in putting up with loneliness, rip-offs of every kind and boredom, and able to live on a pittance. He or she, although not demented, which would be a nuisance to other people, is slightly deficient in intellect and tiresome to talk to, because folklore says that old people are weak in the head, asexual, because old people are incapable of sexual activity, and it is unseemingly if they are not. He or she is unemployable, because old age is second childhood and everyone knows that the old make a mess of simple work. Some credit points can be gained by visiting or by being nice to a few of these subhuman individuals, but most of them prefer their own company and the company of other aged unfortunates. Their main occupations are religion, grumbling, reminiscing and attending the funerals of friends. If sick, they need not, and should not, be actively treated, and are best stored in unsupervised institutions run by racketeers who fleece them and hasten their demise. A few, who are amusing or active, are kept by society as pets. The rest are displaying unpardonable bad manners by continuing to live, and even on occasion by complaining of their treatment, when society has declared them unpeople and their patriotic duty is to lie down and die.[4]

The wonderful thing I have found in geriatric health education and nursing is that this stereotype is a myth. For increasing numbers of older people, their later years are a time for the growth and personal development for which they never had time in their busy younger years. I've always wondered why texts on growth and development focus on pediatrics. Current psychological research confirms the fact that many older people achieve new levels of creativity and insight with advancing years. W. Somerset Maugham puts it very well when he states:

> When I was young I was amazed at Plutarch's statement that the older Cato began at the age of eighty to learn Greek. I am amazed no longer. Old age is ready to undertake tasks that youth shirked because they would take too long.

It is surprising to many health professionals how well older persons often respond to treatment and learn self-care. There's a notion that old age is characterized by inevitable and irreversible degeneration requiring nursing care for minimal maintenance and comfort. Not true. If anything, retirement often gives people the time to take care of themselves in ways they've never had time for before.

Members of the health education clubs, Senior Health Source, sponsored by the Albuquerque Bernalillo County Office of Senior Affairs, are one example of groups that have taken responsibility for their health in holistic ways. At weekly meetings groups of adults from 55 to 95 years of age meet to re-create the concepts originated in the ancient Egyptian Temple Beautiful. The focus is on ways to regain personal-life-power and to learn to create and share energy among the group members. Members first use meditation, biofeedback, and visualization techniques to go inside and re-create a true love of their bodies and appreciation for the miracle of the life processes. Then they work with enlarging and moving energy into and out of their bodies to heal themselves and those they care for. Reflexology, Therapeutic Touch, taking each others' blood pressure, and observing biorhythms are some of the simple ways for group members to use energy fields and natural healing power. Once older persons regain a feeling of power over being able to influence their own physical condition, they usually reach out to help others.

Unfortunately we are working with a disease model of care. There is much to overcome in creating holistic attitudes. When a person receives a diagnosis, he or she is told all the horrible complications and side-effects that are possible or probable. Clearly, part of medical education is how to communicate realistically with our patients as to what their true prognosis is. There is also much to be said about self-fulfilling prophesies. What about the person who refuses to believe he or she will never walk again and goes on to prove it by walking? What is there to prevent us from also including love, the power of positive visualization, spiritual healing, or miracles in our prognosis?

What we have created among many older people is a population of "worried well." Sidney Garfield, founder of the Kaiser Permanente Hospitals, postulates that 30% to 50% of all patients entering a physician's office are concerned about their health and essentially are seeking reassurance about their health, which is basically normal. In reality, it's not good for business to encourage and educate patients to care for themselves. Many physicians become wealthy on the $25.00 office visits of elderly Medicaid patients to get their blood pressures checked weekly by a nurse. Unfortunately, many health providers are also aware of the role they play in elderly women's lives as surrogate husbands, sons, or lovers. The physician may be the only man who ever physically touches a 70-year-old widow who lives alone. This widow may even go to the beauty shop before every visit to the physician, and she may wear her prettiest dress. Then she is kept waiting for two hours, sees her physician hurriedly for 10 minutes, and gets answers to none of her questions. Clearly not all medical practitioners are so callous; however, testimony speaks for itself. Just as Medicare/Medicaid provides for much needed care and treatment of older persons, it can also be highly abused.

I recall an older woman who shared with me how on her 65th birthday her podiatrist sent her a birthday card with her montly appointment reminder. Upon visiting him, he asked her if she wasn't now eligible for Medicare/Medicaid to pay her bill? This hadn't occurred to her, but she checked and found that she was eligible. The podiatrist then congratulated her on not having to pay the bills any longer herself. The woman came to me when she received a duplicate copy of the bill her podiatrist submitted to Medicare for payment. Now that the government was paying, he had raised his fee from $12.00 to $28.00 for the treatment. When I offered to help her report the obvious abuse, she refused because she didn't want to have to find another doctor; however, her feelings toward him were forever changed and her problems with her feet worsened.

The challenge for nurses and health educators is to help the older person feel like a more powerful participant in the process of health care.

We encourage people to write down all their questions on a piece of paper and not to leave until they show them to the doctor. After a session in our health clubs talking about how to ask good questions, someone shared that her physician charged her double because he had to spend extra time talking. Another told of a physician who became enraged when his 82-year-old hypertensive patient refused to leave until he rewrote his Lanoxin prescription so she could read it. The patient wanted to shop around the discount drugstores in town for the cheapest price and needed to be able to tell the pharmacists over the phone what she was shopping for. The enraged physician ended up having his nurse type out the prescription. The patient ended up finding a more cooperative physician.

This sense of personal worth, self-control, and responsibility has been identified by Abraham Maslow in his *Hierarchy of Human Needs* as one of the essential needs of humans. The holistic health nurse can respond to this new image of aging and can overcome the ambivalence and stereotyping that have characterized the care of older people in the past. He or she can join an enlarging health team that realizes the problems of aging are not without solutions and that older persons themselves have a true depth of experience and rich inner resources to call upon if they are only given the chance. The willingness to explore new attitudes toward the body and new methods of self-care need not be relegated to the affluent, educated young.

Cultural Views of Older Persons

Once a nurse overcomes the stereotypes and recognizes the very special individuality of each older person, he or she needs to push a little deeper and become aware of cultural influences. This is true where I work in the Southwestern United States where Native Americans share the area with Anglo-Saxons and *personas Espanol*. Probed carefully, almost every geographic area, whether urban or rural, has inhabitants with roots in some ethnic origins, be it Oriental, Eastern European, or Latin American.

The values and attitudes that come from these roots are very important to the older persons. The fact that many of our patients today were immigrants at the turn of the century is not always apparent, and many older persons have learned to guard their innermost ways of being because they may have experienced ridicule for their old-fashioned ways. As we become more holistic we are coming to understand and place a new value on cultural differences. To help a person who is experiencing illness or to teach someone how to maintain good health both require being able to speak to the place where that person is willing to hear. All too often patient teaching is done for the benefit of the teacher, and the student comes away with nothing more than when he began or, worse, a feeling of inadequacy. Primary to influencing health behavior is the awareness of when the patient is ready to learn and, more importantly, being able to go to the patient's level of understanding and orientation and begin from there. Often it soon becomes apparent that it is the patient who has something to teach the nurse.

Once nurses are clear in their own minds of how they feel toward people from different races or cultures, they can push through to their role as patient advocate and help their patients overcome the prejudice that is constantly there. Working in public health, the nurse sooner or later must confront both racism and agism. Alex Comfort says agism and racism resemble each other. He sees agism as based on fear, folklore, and the hang-ups of a few unlovable people who propagate it. Like racism, agism needs to be met by information, contradiction, and, when necessary, confrontation. It helps to understand that when societies mistreat a particular group, they usually do it out of fear. We mistreat older patients because we fear our own aging. We mistreat ethnic minorities because their differences challenge our security in our own ways.

It's very exciting to see the role holistic health is playing in opening once-closed doors between cultural groups and encouraging a new communication. The Medical School of the University of New Mexico has opened a branch campus on the Navajo reservation where

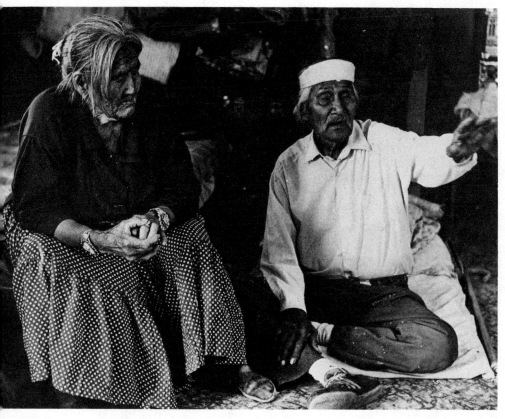

Fig. 16–2.
Elderly Navajo couple. The husband is blind and suffers from Parkinson's disease. His wife nurses him in a one-room hogan on the reservation. *(Photo by Abigail Adler)*

medical students and physicians share a clinic with local tribal medicine men. When the ministrations of one don't work, the other is consulted. Once each year the Kayenta-based Cancer Control Program sponsors a medicine man's retreat where physicians and Navajo medicine men go away for three days together to trade notes.

Natural healing among Spanish-heritage people, as perpetuated by the curanderisimo traditions, is shared in rural health clinics. The natural bounty of nature's herbs is part of the daily practice of preventive medicine promoted by the Curandera in many small Spanish communities. As we become aware of the value of these practices, the native practitioners become more willing to share them for responsible use. All around the country there is a growing appreciation for natural therapeutics that have been in use, often secretly, for generations.

When older persons realize that they will not be ridiculed for

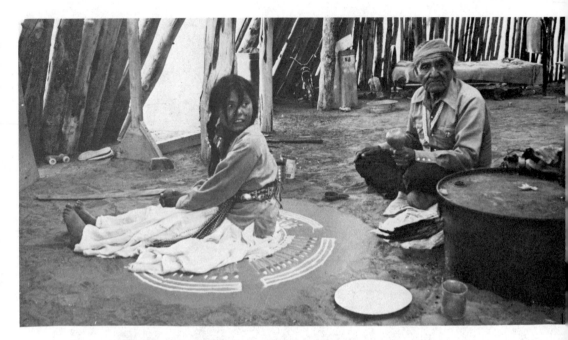

Fig. 16–3.
A Navajo medicine man performs an ancient sand painting healing on a young girl. *(Photo by Abigail Adler)*

practicing an age-old custom, they are more willing to share what they're doing for their condition and the nurse is better able to make an assessment for intervention, knowing the whole situation. Often the old and the new can be combined, as in the case of an elderly arthritic who refused to come into the clinic for hydrotherapy but agreed to use hot paraffin at home for swollen knuckles and fingers. Someone who cannot remember to take Digoxin every morning can be encouraged to take it with a morning dose of lemon and honey, which is never forgotten.

As professionals we have to maintain a healthy skepticism concerning alternative health practices, but I would hope we can also understand that what may appear worthless therapy to one could have dynamic results for the person who believes in it. Much of medicine is ritual. Who is to say that white coats are any less a ritual costume than colored feathers?

Becoming aware of other cultural attitudes is a true growth opportunity. I never understood how much I had "bought in" to efficiency and cost-effective clinic care until I was privileged to attend several Native American healing rituals. There, time is an endless quantity. To begin the ceremony at the right time is crucial, and only the medicine man knows when that is. Everyone waits, patiently into the night, next morning, or days later. This sense of being patient for the correct elements to be in place is difficult for my capitalistic, Anglo-Saxon efficiency orientation. But if I hope to be able to help these people with their health needs, I had better learn to wait.

In caring for Spanish-heritage older persons I have come to understand and not be critical of those who refuse to admit they are ill and seek help. Macho is real. An 82-year-old patriarch will not admit to having crushing chest pains because it would be a sign of weakness, and he is strong. Much as I disagree with his need to act that way, it is his self-concept and I have no right to pass judgment. I do have an obligation for some inspired health teaching.

Perhaps the most difficult cultural attitude I have to accept has led me to my area of greatest challenge. I am speaking of the individual's right to determine when and where his own death will occur. Throughout history ethnologists have documented this custom among native peoples. Elderly Eskimos say their goodbyes, pack their kayaks, and float into the Arctic sea. Among the Hopi, the Creek, and the Crow, it was once customary to lead the aged person to a specially built hut away from the village and there leave him, according to his own wishes, with little food or water, to die. One cannot help wonder if the current trend in the care of terminally ill patients, the *Hospice* concept, is not a connection with an ancient archetype of the individual choreographing his or her own death. Our's is the privilege to consciously witness and honor another's passing.

We are trained to help people recover and get better. Often health providers take it very personally and feel they have failed when that doesn't happen. Essential to allowing a person to be whole in living is the necessity to let the person go when he or she is ready. It is very difficult to continue nursing someone who is slowly failing and leaving. (We may even feel it is time wasted. We could be helping someone who will recover.) If we are truly to see our patients as whole, we must also allow them power in their dying and honor their final wishes, even if it means hastening their deaths by not providing all the modern technology we know could keep them alive longer. It is their choice, their final choice.

Nursing Process: View of Our Own Aging

Part of becoming a holistic health nurse includes a new view of ourselves as individuals and as professionals. My wish would be that we not be frightened to look in the faces of very old people and see ourselves. Can we keep our sense of humor about the critical scrutiny for each new wrinkle, blemish, or change with age that goes on in front of the mirror each morning? I am reminded of a poem by a 76-year-old woman entitled "Ode to Raging Wrinkles." She was thanking God she didn't have to worry about what she looked like anymore. She could save all the money she used to spend on creams, lotions, and beauty potions, and use the money to take a trip to Spain.

We live in a commercial marketplace determined to sell us everything we could ever need to maintain our youthful selves. It's a billion-dollar industry. To remain handsome, ageless, and alluring is a sign of great status in our society. Our self-concepts are closely tied to our physical presentation. It is a common fear that when you lose your looks you lose your appeal and nobody will be attracted to you ever again.

As nurses we confront the veritable search for the fountain of youth when the traveler goes astray. There are any number of unseemly characters out to defraud the aging (of all ages) with potentially dangerous products that are guaranteed to renew their energy, youth, and beauty. This is not only a financial injustice for people on fixed incomes, but it can also bring our patients into clinics with severe side-effects. I recall one elderly gentleman who gave himself scalp cancer with some magic remedy that also required he spend several hours per day in the direct sunlight. It may not have been dangerous in the rainy Northwest, but in New Mexico he severely damaged his skin. When it was announced that certain hair dyes were suspected of causing skin cancer, the Senior Health Source health clubs had long talks about our emotional attachments to our hair and what it felt like when it started thinning and turning grey. Maggie Kuhn of the Grey Panthers has done more than anyone to destigmatize the coming of the grey in people's lives.

As nurses we are taught the careful scrutiny of our patients' bodies. We delve into their most private lives and look around. Are we as willing to take a long look at ourselves? Can we stand naked in front of a mirror and really see who we are and take responsibility for change, if need be? Can we really influence our diabetic patients to lose weight if we're bursting our own seams? Do we need yoga or meditation to offset the stress that creeps into our posture and disposition? Perhaps the question to ask is: "What am I a model of? What do I inspire by my way of being in the world? Can I help my menopausal patient adjust to her aging process when I'm terrified of my own fortieth birthday?"

Nurses as Guides and Teachers

Nursing is an ancient profession, extending over time from tribal shamanism to the American Nurses Association. People involved with healing set themselves apart by taking responsibility for being prepared to offer a service others can trust. Years of training and preparation provide a basis for giving care and being accountable. The commitment to become holistic, to care for the whole person, also requires bringing our whole selves to the task. Unlike other jobs, nursing is not something one hangs up on a peg at the end of the day and leaves behind. Being a nurse is a specific, visible role in the community, and, especially in geriatric nursing, it becomes a part of who you are.

Having once overcome the prejudices against working with the elderly, the holistic nurse can embrace her chosen path and realize she is truly responding to a calling. I like the analogy of the guide. The nurse can see himself or herself as one who has agreed to help others along their path. This is especially true for the public health or home nurse who is the primary member of the health team providing care. Essential to being a guide is the understanding that "when the student is ready, the teacher appears," and that the role of health educator is a privileged one.

We are in the right place at the right time to help someone through a hard time. As the *I Ching* so succinctly tells us, "we must understand the transitory in light of the eternity of the end." We are in a position to influence our patients or students in their journey toward better health. This journey toward health includes our increasing knowledge of the etiology of disease. We are discovering that personality may play a major role in why one person becomes hypertensive and in why another person develops cancer.[5] This vanguard research promises to give us clues as to how we may prevent disease through working with our habits and attitudes—our very ways of being in the world. Unfortunately, it is also fuel to the fire for the "weller than thou" crowd (*i.e.*, "if you weren't so uptight, you wouldn't have heart disease"). A person with a major illness does not need to be blamed for being sick. There is nothing creative about feeling guilty. As helpers and guides to those experiencing major illness, we can allow them to assume responsibility for themselves and their situation without punishing them for not preventing it. You cannot heal something you resent.

As well as being nonjudgmental, a guide is also wide awake on behalf of the patient. Since we have some background in the potential pitfalls and dangers along the way, we have an obligation to pay attention so that we can provide caution when necessary. We can be trusted to be there when we're needed. This may be setting limits. Nothing is harder than firmly communicating with a recent 68-year-old myocardial infarction patient that he will not be able to scale the lofty heights with his son's backpacking club like he once could. Hopefully, he knows and trusts his nurse enough to believe that the nurse is not just trying to scare him but is really his advocate and is sharing a real danger with him.

As well as accepting responsibility to protect the patient, a true guide encourages clients to do as much for themselves as they can. We are not out to create dependency relationships that feed our own egos. We believe in the innate power and ability of each person to manage and create healing in his or her own life, and we support every effort toward self-care and autonomy. If anything, an inspired guide will instill a sense of challenge in others to meet their health obstacles with a feeling of inner strength and confidence that they can succeed, even if in some small way. (Unfortunately, the trend in the care of the aged has been to medicate them so heavily that they can't make demands or perform self-care even if they want to.)

Utmost in a holistic approach is the provision of alternatives. When the door closes, open a window. Nothing works for everyone. Just as everyone is too old for some things, no one is too old for everything. A committed guide does not give up when the underbrush gets heavy. The guide may back off and choose an alternate route, but assures followers that there is a way, and seeks spiritual resources.

When we are educated in specific approaches to complex chronic problems, it is easy to get stuck; and when our traditional methods don't work, it's easy to give up and blame our patient for the patient's inability to learn or cooperate. Perhaps what we really need to do is open ourselves to other alternatives and then be quiet and wait for inspiration. Contrary to popular belief, we found through the Senior Health Source that older persons are open to such widely diverse approaches as reflexology, biofeedback, massage therapy, polarity, shiatzu, Therapeutic Touch, touch for health, and light touch therapy. Often it's the nurse or health care provider rather than the older patient who must be convinced of the viability of a new approach.

Finally, a true guide realizes that he or she doesn't know everything about everything. We are all fallible, and to admit when we don't know the answer is the sign of a good teacher. Often nurses get caught in good intentions and end up creating obstacles for their patients. I recall a student nurse doing a rotation in an adult day care program. She had been alerted to the potential danger to participants who wander out of the building and into the street. All morning she ran resistance to an 88-year-old English woman who repeatedly tried to get out the door to go to Parliament. After the aged lady went to the center supervisor in distress, she was allowed to take her journey. It seems she referred to the toilet as Parliament, and there was the House of Lords for the gentlemen and the House of Commons for the ladies. Perhaps this is also a situation where staff communication is crucial. Older people often create their own realities that are very workable for them. Reality orientation often helps the care provider as much as the patient; at least an agreed reality is created.

Once a nurse agrees to be someone's guide through a time of

aging or ill health, he or she takes on the task of perhaps having to blaze a new trail. Holistic health care is a new orientation for many people, and often the older person cannot articulate to other members of the health team just how he or she wants to be treated. This is where holism comes to its edge and the nurse must expose herself as an advocate for the whole person and not just the person's disease. The nurse must be willing to become vocal, firm, and clear about what the needs of the patient are perceived to be and how the patient would choose to have them met. Hopefully, the nurse is also well educated and persuasive in the effectiveness of alternative methods of care.

Preventive Self-Care and Health Education

The senior health source clubs are just one of many models in a trend among older persons to get together to get healthy. The nurses and health care professionals who coordinate, present programs and classes, and facilitate the flow of information are guides for people who have been attracted to the path of maximizing their personal health. Another excellent model of holistic health for senior citizens is the SAGE project located in Berkeley, California.*

Essentially, self-health involves a focus on health revitalization and maintenance at a high level. It includes the prevention of illness or its recurrence and a continuity of care after sickness within a broad spectrum of alternatives, support systems, and practices.

Perhaps the most valuable aspect of working on personal health within a group is the provision of opportunities to communicate with others about one's deepest worries, fears, or misconceptions, and also developing the skill to actively listen and respond to others. Honest response is very important. Often an older person is merely tolerated as background noise. Some folks think of older persons as "Babylons"; they just babble on and on. Because it is an expectation, some older people get caught up in the sound of their own voice, and their communication does become babble. Even though they are talking all the time, no one is listening, so essentially they are still alone. Self-health groups emphasize meaningful sharing about the here and now and practice becoming aware of meaningful responses to each other. Harvey Jackins has developed an excellent model in his reevaluation counseling therapy:[6] you listen actively to me for an allotted period of time and then I'll listen equally to you. In the clinical or institutional setting, the older person is often overwhelmed and the health team

---

*The SAGE project involves senior actualization and growth explorations. It is located in Berkeley, California, and also includes the headquarters for the National Association for Humanistic Gerontology.

must take time to create a space where the older patient can feel free to share inner questions and feelings. It does not happen naturally; it must be deliberately created and nurtured. And then it must be held in trust. Communication cannot be overemphasized. The health team must remember that not everyone speaks "medicalese." For fear of looking stupid, the older person does not always ask for clarification when confused. One elderly lady was very relieved to discover that when her doctor told her that her Pap test was negative it did not mean that she had cancer. Negative to her had meant bad results. She was waiting to be notified of surgery; she was heartbroken and terrified until told that in this case negative meant good results.

Holistic health education for senior citizens can also provide ways to offset the constant sense of loss an older person faces: loss of physical health or ability; possible loss of spouse, friends, and family; loss of life-long house or home; or loss of hair, sight, teeth, taste, or hearing. The health guide must be considerate of these losses and at the same time maximize the contributions that only a person of age can make to society.

After months in a weekly group meeting, a spunky 80-year-old woman reprimanded the young group leader for turning her back to the group when she spoke. "I didn't see a thing you said" was her criticism. She was stone deaf and had never said a word about it.

A special skill of specific benefit to everyone is teaming the older person up with a child or teenager who needs a foster or surrogate grandparent. When a large city housing site for seniors adopted a preschool for emotionally handicapped children, no one imagined the benefit that would accrue all the way around. Perhaps the most important sharing was tactile. Here were two groups of individuals who were not receiving enough physical contact. The cuddling and fondling that occurred at group sessions with the children opened doors to allow the seniors to touch each other more readily. Too often the older person is not hugged or embraced by others because he or she seems fragile or easily knocked off center. This is true. However, someone living alone needs nonverbal, physical communication from others when part of a group. Simply holding someone's hand or putting an arm around a shoulder may be the only physical contact that person has had for days or weeks. Physical isolation is a reality of aging in the United States today. Holistic health care providers can help offset its effects by using every contact as an opportunity to touch that person in as many ways as possible.

Self-health education includes providing opportunities for older persons to become more self-sufficient and self-reliant. At a time in their lives when they are expected to accept help with an increasingly large number of things that they could once do alone, it feels good to have a little power in one's life. Growing one's own green vegetable seeds in a Mason jar for sprouting or making skinlotions in the blender

is not only cost-effective but also allows the older persons to provide
something for themselves. The organization of food clubs to buy staples
in bulk from local co-ops gave senior citizens an opportunity to not pay
the high prices at the local chain store. Clearly, individuals on fixed
incomes are most vulnerable to inflation, and every effort to provide
financial relief is appreciated. One group of elderly persons organized a
solar energy organization to build themselves a solar greenhouse so
they could start their garden vegetables early in the spring. Simple,
basic health maintenance begins with a good long look at the available
resources within a community that provide opportunities for senior
citizens to do for themselves. A local women's health collective
responded to a need and trained volunteers to act as "health advocates"
and go with an older woman to her physician or clinic and provide a
support system for her to ask for and receive the care she wanted.

Essentially, the role of holistic health for senior citizens goes
beyond communication, contact, and power, to promoting a sense of
excitement about fully experiencing this sunset time of life.
Overcoming society's sense of inertia associated with aging is a major
feat. This can be a time of incredible growth and development if the
expectation of that occurring is created. For the members of the health
team, working with self-actualized older persons is a chance to create a
positive expectation of their own aging, as well as to share in the fun.

Holistic Health Education Allies

Medical education goes to great lengths to emphasize the importance of
teamwork in caring for people's complex human needs. Systems have
been developed to standardize our responses so that continuity of care
can be provided. One of these is the Problem-Oriented Medical Records
(POMR) system. It assures that the individual is seen in terms of the
priorities of his or her problems. In an acute situation, this is very
valuable. In a holistic atmosphere of care, could we not rewrite the
system to provide Person-Oriented Medical Responses?

The person-oriented system includes all the possible resources
within the community that respond to any of the individual's needs.
This means interagency contact and coordination for care.
Transportation, housing, nutrition, homemaker help, visiting nursing
service, and spiritual and mental outreach may all be needed.
Unfortunately, health care is a multibillion-dollar industry, and all too
often agencies and institutions look upon their patients as paying
customers; they become possessive of their needs and treat them like
"turf" to be guarded and jealously hoarded, especially if Medicare or
Medicaid is paying the bill. Hopefully, the holistic orientation will pave
the way for the emphasis to go back on the individual concerned, and

all those involved will recognize who most effectively provides what is needed.

There do exist many high-intentioned organizations and groups that provide excellent back-up services to the health team. Church auxiliaries provide transportation and friendly visits and telephone calls. Boy Scouts and Girl Scouts give generously of their time to entertain and visit with older, hospitalized persons. National organizations such as the Heart, Diabetes, and Cancer Associations provide resource materials, speakers, films, and often special services for specific problems. The Lion's Club has given itself a mandate to help those who have lost their sight, and even sent an elderly gentleman to the Midwest to receive a seeing-eye dog. There are many individuals in every community who respond to the natural human urge to give of themselves. They simply need a place to plug in, a person to help.

The nurse should remember all her allies when she becomes frustrated for options in the care of an elderly patient. We are not in this alone, and just as our patients and students need support and reassurance, so do we. It's o.k. to feel overwhelmed. Perhaps one of the most difficult lessons for a care-giver to learn is how to receive, how to ask for help and accept it. Natural networks of caring individuals are real. The creation of a network of holistic health nurses will allow individual nurses to expand their ability to provide for their patients and enlarge their repertoire of alternatives that they can make available to the patients and to themselves.

On the most personal level, each individual nurse has his or her own guides and teachers. If we are to guide our patients through the rapids of illness on their rivers of life, we will need to provide nourishment and inspiration for ourselves when we are in insecure or troubled waters. This is a new age and there are many new sources of information and motivation. An open mind and a willingness to try new ways of thinking or feeling are basic elements of holism. Perhaps our best teachers are our patients and the reflection of ourselves we see in them. Certainly in gerontology and work with senior citizens, the nurse is provided with an opportunity to receive from those who have endured the tests of time and come out smiling.

Experiential Exercise

1. Old age simulation. In working with older persons, it is of value to attempt to "step into their shoes." This is done with the help of a few essential props:
   a. Place damp cotton balls in both ears to decrease hearing.
   b. Hold a marble under your tongue to simulate ill-fitting dentures.
   c. Wrap crumpled plastic wrap around your eyes to create blurred vision as with glaucoma or cataracts.

    d. Tie a splint on one knee to create an immobile arthritic joint.

    e. Place a glove on your right hand and insert small wooden pencils in at least two fingers to simulate arthritis.

Now walk up and down unfamiliar stairs. Read the small print on a food label. Write your name in a limited space and thread a needle. Talk on the telephone. Try to appreciate the limitations an older person lives with.

2. Sit quietly and breathe deeply while you progress yourself up in age. Can you actively image yourself at the age of 50, then 60, then 70 and 80. Carefully create what you will look like. What do you project your major health problems will be? How will your disposition and personality age? Where will you be living and how much money will you have to get by? What kind of relationship will you have with your family and what kind of friends will you have?

3. Think of five things you are planning to accomplish during your lifetime.

    a. Eliminate the one you will be unable to do if you lose your vision.

    b. Eliminate the one you cannot do if you develop crippling arthritis.

    c. You have just been informed that your prognosis is to live one more year. Prioritize your time. What would you do with your remaining days?

    d. Consider your feelings if you were 76 years old and were unable to achieve any of your goals due to circumstances beyond your control.

References

1. Comfort A: A Good Age, p 22. New York, Simon & Schuster, 1976
2. Hess P, Day C: Understanding the Aging Patient, p 17. Bowie, Md, Robert J Brady, 1977
3. Burnside IM: Nursing and the Aged, p 10. New York, McGraw-Hill, 1976
4. Comfort, *ibid*, p 23
5. Pelletier K: Mind as Healer, Mind as Slayer. New York, Dell, 1977
6. Jackins H: The Human Situation. Seattle, Rational Island Publishers, 1973

Suggested Readings

Beck PV, Walters AL: The Sacred. Tsalie, Arizona, Navajo Community College Press, 1977

Burnside IM: Nursing and the Aged. New York, McGraw-Hill, 1976

Butler RN, Lewis MI: Aging and Mental Health, 2nd ed. St Louis, CV Mosby, 1977

Comfort A: A Good Age. New York, Simon & Schuster, 1976

Curtin SR: Nobody Ever Died of Old Age. Boston, Little, Brown, 1972

de Beauvoir S: The Coming of Age. New York, GP Putnam's Sons, 1970

Fann WE, Madox G: Drug Issues in Geropsychiatry. Baltimore, Williams & Wilkins, 1974

Hess P, Day C: Understanding the Aging Patient. Bowie, Md, Robert J Brady, 1977

Jackins H: The Human Situation. Seattle, Rational Island Publishers, 1973

Pelletier K: Mind as Healer, Mind as Slayer. New York, Dell, 1977

17 Death: A Natural Facet of the Life Continuum

Cathleen A. Fanslow

It is essential that any text on holistic health for nurses include sections on all of life, including death as part of the continuum of life. The first general principle influencing the study of death is its normalcy, that is, the fact that "death is a part of life."

Nursing students must be given the knowledge and clinical tools to deal with dying persons and their families just as they are taught the care of the mother and the child during birth. Both birth and death are normal and natural processes. Since we know that prenatal care has a decided effect on the healthy life and delivery of the infant, so too realistic and effective predeath preparation of both patient and family has a decided effect on the "healthy" death of the patient.

Historical Perspective

Early birth practices in all cultures were truly natural and holistic, with the mother performing her normal tasks up until the moment of delivery. Our history is filled with the normalcy of birth, of children born in cotton fields, wheat fields, Conestoga wagons, log cabins, and in cities and towns as well as en route to the West. With the incursion of medical technology, some of the naturalness of the process was lost, being replaced by sterile delivery rooms and anesthesia. While these innovations have markedly decreased the infant mortality rate, the birth trauma has been increased.

In order to reestablish the balance in the birth process and restore normalcy to the beginning of the life continuum, natural childbirth methods such as Lamaze, Leboyer, and others have come into fashion. These methods stress the naturalness of the delivery of the child and attempt to normalize the environment into which the child enters. As a result, the birth trauma is lessened, the child breathes more quickly, and both parents spontaneously and actively participate in beginning this new individual's life journey in a more natural way, unencumbered by drugs, resuscitation, or forceps. The parents and others assisting at the birth become present to the infant in a very real and natural way.

The external manifestation of the unique presence of the child's parents at this time is signified by the placing of the newborn child on the mother's abdomen or by putting the child to her breast minutes after birth. The beginning of the trust relationship between primary care-giver and child is manifested by the circle made by the mother's and father's arms as the child lies nestled in them, secure in this beginning of a new life.

It has been necessary to discuss by means of a historical perspective the return to normalcy of the birth process in order to stress the need for a return to the naturalness and normalcy of the dying process because this too has undergone many changes.

In the past in all cultures, the ceremonies surrounding death and the nursing and the care of the dying were all part of daily living. The aged and ill were kept at home as an integral part of the extended family. They died in the arms of family members, were waked in the parlor, and were buried in many cases from the houses in which they had come into the world.

With the advent of the Industrial Revolution and increased mobility, the bonds of the extended family were severed. The result was that care of the dying and death itself no longer took place in the family home, but were relegated to the alien environment of nursing home or hospital.

It is unrealistic to think that we will be able to return to the time of the extended family structure, when the naturalness of the death process was considered part of everyday life. It becomes even more imperative that those who comprise the "new family" of the dying person in the foreign environment of the hospital or nursing home be given the knowledge and clinical tools to create an environment wherein the dying person is assisted to die in a natural and normal way. Due to our advanced technology, the creation and maintenance of such a natural humanistic milieu become the primary role of the final care-giver, who in most instances is the nurse. The approach must be that death is indeed a part of life, an integral part of the wellness spectrum. Indeed, one might say that death is the completion of life itself—its holistic completion.

The Nurse–Practitioner's Awareness

In order to effectively relate to dying persons and their families, it is absolutely essential that nurse–practitioners become aware of their own attitudes, feelings, and fears concerning death, which affect their interaction with the dying, and how to deal with them in a natural and holistic manner.

Beginning nurse–practitioners must be assisted in a gentle but real manner to take an inward journey where they are challenged to look at those factors that have contributed to the formation of not only their own philosophy of life but also their philosophy of death. Early death experiences and their effect on the nursing student need to be investigated and clarified because they are the cornerstones of developing attitudes and fears of death. In this area more than in any other it is imperative that nurses become consciously aware of who they are and who they can become, for themselves as well as for their dying patients and families.

Just as there are general principles that govern the laws of nature and the universe, there are also many principles that govern our attitude and approach to the dying. The principles directly related to the dying process itself are the following:

1. The first general principle influencing and affecting any member of the health-care system who will relate to the dying is the fact that "death is a part of life." A moment of honest reflection will tell us that in the natural order of all life, both the living and the dying are inclusive of one another; that death is actually a part of life, the completion of the life process itself.

2. The second general principle affecting the students' study of death as well as their interaction with the dying is the fact of our own mortality, that one day we too will die, as all other living creatures will die. This fact, by its universality, creates a bond between us and the dying and has helped care-givers numerous times when confronted or challenged by a dying person. In those difficult moments, attempts to tune into the fact that we too will die like the person before us helps us respond to what that person is asking of us—to help that person die as he or she wishes.

3. The third very important yet often unspoken principle that greatly affects our interaction with the dying person is our fear of our own death. The most basic fear surrounding death appears to be the fear of the unknown, and like the second principle, it possesses a universal quality. Again, when seemingly at a loss for words of comfort in the face of impending death, an acknowledgment of fear of the unknown such as "it's scary to be so sick" or "this sure is a frightening experience, isn't it" can enable one to link up with the universal principle of fear of death, fear of the unknown, and support the dying person from a totally human, fully shared, and natural and holistic perspective.

Integration of these three basic principles into the practitioner's life as well as into his or her philosophy of death will indeed help the Renaissance Nurse's personal evolution as well as enable this nurse to intervene more realistically and effectively with dying persons and their families.

With the three general principles forming the foundation of the holistic study of death as the culmination of the living process, let us now turn our attention to what is needed in order to return this fact of life called death to its natural place in the dying patient's life continuum.

As we examine our two most basic needs as living persons, we conclude that they are also the two most basic needs of dying persons. The two basic needs of dying persons are the following: (1) they need to know that they will never be abandoned and (2) they have a need for hope.

We attend to the first basic need of dying patients by establishing and maintaining a trust relationship with them. The trust comes from the nurse–practitioner's desire to care for them in the most real and sensitive manner of which he or she is capable, that is, using the whole self in the most natural holistic way possible. The holistic self has been brought forth by means of the examination of past death experiences, current searching and discussion of death and dying, as well as by the development of a philosophy of death that is experiential.

Our contact, be it visual, verbal, emotional, or psychological, is part of our contract with persons approaching the end of the life continuum. They need to know that they will not be abandoned. Persons in the last stage of life can't tolerate a moment of uncertainty. They can't be left to wonder "where," "how," "when," and "if" you will actualize your promise to them. Assurance that this basic need will be taken care of eradicates their basic fear of abandonment.

Realistically, we know very well that we cannot always be "with" our dying patients. It is the quality of the presence of the care-giver, not the quantity of time spent, that actualizes the contract. An important point to bear in mind is that trusting is not synonymous with knowing all the answers. The nurse–practitioner doesn't have to say anything or be afraid of saying "the wrong thing"; he or she just has to be.

This "being" is achieved from the experiential study described later in the text. This method enables student nurses to "become" in touch with themselves and their philosophy of the life–death continuum. This self-knowing on a very deep level of their own attitudes, feelings, and fears of the death process enables them to hear the attitudes, feelings, and fears of their patients. Once health-care professionals have been sensitized through self-awareness to what their own philosophy on death is, and once they are somewhat grounded in that knowledge, they can then listen objectively, *and truly hear what* the patient is saying about this most important fact of life.

As beginning professionals, they will have to accept, or at least acknowledge on some level, that they cannot stop the cancer or progressive chronic illness. They are unable to announce to the patient in a reassuring manner that the treatments have stopped the disease process.

When the dying person persists in reminding us that death has supreme power over us, we suddenly are made to feel hopeless and helpless. To alleviate the guilt feelings that this state of hopelessness provokes in us, we then direct our energies toward those who have hope for life, only because we view death as a personal failure. Thus we further isolate dying patients, nonverbally communicating to them that they are bad for not allowing us to be victorious over death. They symbolize our frustration. To face them is to face that we too are mortal. As we have shared life, so too shall we share death.

Support in Hope

The person with the knowledge of impending death is literally dying for hope. As professionals we are faced with the responsibility to support our terminal patients in their hopes. How can we do this when we know that death is approaching? How can we offer this support without lying to the patient, thus betraying our trust relationship? The only way we can effectively communicate this is by eliciting from the patient the object of his hope. Anyone can live with the fact that he has an incurable disease, but no one can live with the thought that he, as a person, is hopeless. Since hope is of the very essence of human life, humans would die without it. Therefore, hope is most necessary for dying persons because it enables them to live each day until they die.

As a result of my own clinical experience, I have developed a four-phase system, useful in keeping hope alive in the dying person. This system, which is simply called the *Hope System*, describes how the nature of hope changes in persons in the final stage of the life continuum. It motivates them to live through the dying process from the moment of the diagnosis of the fatal disease or condition until death itself.

Initially the patient experiences phase one, Hope for Cure (*e.g.*, "I hope I only have infectious mononucleosis or hepatitis and *not* leukemia"). As time passes, the patient moves to phase two, where Hope for Treatment predominates over the initial Hope for Cure (*e.g.*, "I have a tumor [growth], and the radiation will shrink it and I will be all right again"). Thirdly, when faced with the prospect that "there is nothing more that we (the medical world) can do for you," the patient's hope turns to Hope for Prolongation of Life (*e.g.*, "I hope to live longer, for in time they will find a cure"). Finally, when the dying patient no longer hopes for life and is able to let go of that to which he clings so frantically, he moves to the final phase, where Hope for a Peaceful Death predominates.

The health professional must determine which phase of the Hope System predominates for the patient at any given time. Once this is ascertained, it is the responsibility of the care-giver to provide the patient with the supportive care needed during that phase. Encouragement, information, and understanding of the diagnosis and treatment are essential during Hope for Cure and Hope for Treatment, as opposed to the comfort, care, palliation, and presence needed during the Hope for a Peaceful Death phase. It must be clear to the professional that the patient's hope may not be the same hope that the professional has for him at that time. Support of the patient's Hope System is always our priority, for this hope is his reality. By utilizing the Hope System as a frame of reference as well as by responding to the basic needs of the dying person we can more meaningfully accompany the patient on his final journey and assist him to die well.

The predominant hope or thrust in the first phase of the Hope System is the Hope for Cure (*i.e.*, "whatever I have is curable; let it be only anemia or infectious mononucleosis. I don't have leukemia, multiple sclerosis, or a disease that is incurable"). This theme may recede to the background as other phases move into the most predominant spot; however, it is always present in the first three phases within the patient and affects his perception of his reality. The Hope for Cure phase is closely allied with the stage of initial denial, shock, and disbelief of Dr. Elisabeth Kübler-Ross.[1] Because the predominant hope is for cure, one often hears patients say, after hearing the diagnosis, that they have a tumor, a growth, a blood disease, a lump, or so on. They do not say the word *cancer* or *malignancy*. Uttering the dreaded word may validate the fact that they do have something that ultimately cannot be cured, because on some internal level, cancer, the word itself, means that what one has is incurable. The thought of having something incurable is a pattern inconsistent with the fundamental hope for cure, so the thought is pushed to the background. This phenomenon enables patients to react from the shock of the initial diagnosis and prognosis and marshall their own internal forces.

As time passes, the major thrust of the Hope System, while anchored in Hope for Cure, moves into the second phase where the predominant hope seems to be placed in the treatment modalities prescribed for the patient. For example, "I have a lump and the doctor will remove it surgically and everything will be all right"; or "Me and the cobalt are gonna beat this thing"; or "There's a new medicine the doctor will give into my vein and it will take care of my blood problem." In this phase, one sees and hears patients and families place their hope in new equipment or medications. They are still, as befits our human condition, hoping for cure, but now it is expressed in the hope that the treatment will effect a cure. I compare this second phase to the anger stage of Dr. Elisabeth Kübler-Ross. This phase usually finds the patient undergoing a variety of strenuous therapeutic modalities that require a great deal of energy. In reality, the Hope for Treatment phase utilizes the anger the patient is experiencing in a positive manner, thus actually sustaining him through the treatments.

In the third phase, the predominant hope is Hope for Prolongation of Life and becomes activated when the person is told, after enduring the treatment regimens, that "there is nothing more that we in medical science can do for you." Hope for Prolongation of Life can be considered comparable to bargaining, the third of Dr. Kübler-Ross's stages. Dying persons hope for prolongation of life; essentially they hope for time, because time can grant the miracle and find a cure.

This hope is strengthened and becomes operant in the face of the admission by those in the medical world that they have done their utmost. When confronted by this stark fact, the persons hold on even more tightly to what is known; that is, they hold onto life. The Hope for Prolongation of Life becomes most strong and is maintained for a very long period, particularly by the parents of dying children and adolescents. This occurs because the thought of children dying, or going to "non-life" and leaving the parents, is so against nature's laws and therefore overwhelming to comprehend and accept.

The fourth phase of the hope system is the Hope for a Peaceful Death. Here, the underlying hope is no longer for cure but rather for a death that is peaceful. The term *peaceful* is more comprehensive than terms such as *painless, quick,* and so on, because it implies freedom not only from physical pain but also from emotional and spiritual pain, and, even more crucial, freedom from mental anguish. The movement from Hope for Prolongation of Life to Hope for a Peaceful Death is signified by a behavioral change unique to each person. There is a letting go of the things of this life and of relationships, particularly relationships that have a special meaning to the dying person, such as his own significant others.

Withdrawal, rejection, going inward, sleeping more, and verbalizing less signify that the person is beginning the last leg of his earthly journey, and our responsibility here is to assist him in achieving his last hope for death that is peaceful on all levels. The last phase of the Hope System may be likened to the acceptance phase of the dying process as described by Dr. Kübler-Ross, "since the componant of peace is contained in both approaches."

The clinical application of this tool has proved effective and has provided a language and a system to better understand and interact with dying persons and their families. I feel it is crucial for those of us interacting with dying persons because it enables us to get at the heart of the matter. That is, it helps us understand what the dying person is truly hoping for from this experience, this treatment, this surgery, this hospitalization. Thus it helps us picture what both life and death mean for this person.

It has been said that we are what we hope for. In this, the final life crisis, how much more effective we will be if we elicit what our patients and their families are hoping for. As in any effective, meaningful, therapeutic interaction, it is essential that health professionals be exquisitely aware of their own hope systems in relationship to their own patients. They must honestly and consistently confront themselves and ask what it is they are hoping for this patient at this point in time. This honest self-evaluation and confrontation are essential to the establishing and maintaining of an effective therapeutic relationship.

If health-care practitioners are not clear in what they hope for their patients, they will not be able to hear what the patients are hoping for themselves. Care-givers will not ask the necessary questions, assuming they know the Hope System of their patients, and this is where the danger lies.

If we are uncertain or unclear or hesitant about out Hope System, we are not open to respond to the Hope Systems of our patients. There is the danger that we will impose our own hope system on them because of our own uncertainty. The prime responsibility is never to impose our own Hope System on a patient but rather to be the swing person, free to move because we are grounded in our own knowledge. The health professional is then free to move to whatever phase of the hope system the patient is in and give him the support needed to deal with that phase.

Perhaps a clinical example will elucidate this for you. Mr. F., a patient of mine, had been readmitted to the head and neck service, and he requested that I come to see him. Mr. F. had had five prior admissions in 2½ years, and when last discharged he had a permanent tracheotomy and feeding tube, and to all intents and purposes that had been his last admission. My predominant hope based on my previous experiences with Mr. F. and his last hospitalization was Hope for a Peaceful Death; Mr. F. had been through so much and in my mind had suffered enough.

To my surprise, an elated, animated, though weakened man greeted me. In a lively manner he began to describe a new surgery the doctor was going to try that perhaps would enable him to be rid of the feeding tube at last. He then was taken down to the radiology department, which gave me time to reflect and reexamine my own feelings. In order to be effective in this or any therapeutic trust relationship, it was necessary for me to be clear on my own Hope System, which was affected by my knowledge, intuition, diagnosis, clinical experience, and, of course, my feeling for the patient.

First, I had to be clear in what I had hoped for Mr. F. In all honesty, I was still hoping for a peaceful death for him. But what was his predominant hope? Certainly Hope for Treatment predominated, with underlying Hope for Cure and very much, for now at least, Hope for Prolongation of Life to have the surgery, be rid of the tube, and go home again. Secondly, I had to avoid imposing my Hope for a Peaceful Death on a person whose Hope System was predominantly for life. The support, information, and understanding that this patient required to strengthen his own Hope System at this time were very different from those he would have needed were his predominant hope at the peaceful death phase.

It is the primary responsibility of the health-care professional to elicit and support the hope system of the patient, and this can only be done if he or she first confronts and unearths what he or she hopes for this patient at this time.

The same principle applies in our interaction with the families of the dying in order to give realistic support. We must be very clear on what they hope for their loved ones. Therefore it is essential that the health professional assist and maintain an open communication with the families to elicit and at times help them clarify their Hope System for their loved ones so that they may support them in a more realistic manner.

The Hope System, since it is at the very core of the human person, is an extremely dynamic process which may change frequently. Each new treatment modality, breakthrough, medicine, or piece of equipment may cause it to change. Remember, our Hope System for a patient will also change as we perceive in the patient's clinical, psychological, and emotional state. It is therefore important if this clinical tool, language, and guide are to be effectively utilized that we ascertain as clearly and as honestly as possible what the predominant hope for this patient is at this time. What does he need from us to help him live or die as he hopes for himself, not as we hope for him.

One may think that eliciting a person's Hope System would be very difficult to accomplish. However, the opposite appears to be true from my many years of using this approach with patients and families. Actually, it is simple. One has only to ask, "Mr. (or Mrs.) So-and-So, what do you hope for from this surgery (from radiation therapy)?" The fact that you are asking what it is the patient is hoping for imparts to the patient that you are, first, willing to listen to his hope, and, secondly, to accept him as he is, you are also indicating a willingness to enter a trusting relationship wherein the patient becomes free to share on a real and deep level what he is experiencing. This approach, because of its directness, frees the patient from responding in the traditional patient role and establishes a more human interaction where hope can be easily shared and articulated. The response of the patient to this approach is usually given with a sense of relief and is not difficult for him.

Families usually respond in a similar manner; however, they do seem to be somewhat more consistent with their original predominant theme. That is, they maintain Hope for Cure or Hope for Prolongation of Life. They don't appear to fluctuate as much as patients do because they are not continually bombarded by professionals with new treatments, discussion, or possibilities. They respond more to the bond of their relationship with the patient than to changes in the treatment regimen.

The value in using the Hope System as a clinical tool appears to have a dual focus. First, it is effective in helping the nursing staff by enabling them to objectify, identify, and increase their awareness of their own feelings toward death itself and toward dying patients. This inner confrontation allows them to deal more honestly with these feelings and with their patients. Secondly, it facilitates interstaff communication by providing a clinical structure and language which can describe and articulate the nurse-patient interaction. More effective communication between staff and dying persons has and will result from its implementation.

Following is a list of sample exercises to assist the nurse—practitioner in the integration of the Hope System as a useful clinical tool in establishing and maintaining effective, therapeutic relationships with dying patients, families, peer groups, and all members of the health team.

1. Identify and describe the phases of the Hope System.

2. Describe their interaction with the stages of the dying process.

3. Identify the symbolic verbal and nonverbal communication that transpires between family, patient, and staff, thereby demonstrating an increased ability "to listen."

4. Identify the needs of the dying patient and those of the family, utilizing the phases of the Hope System as guidelines. Actual case presentation of current patient and family is the method of choice.

5. Initate staff conferences to share insights and increased awareness of the Hope System in the dying process, thus strengthening peer support and increasing the quality of staff interactions. The staff conference can also be utilized as a forum to introduce the Hope System as an objective language form to describe and understand the dying process and its implications for the staff and the patient.

6. Prepare a patient care plan, reflecting an understanding of the Hope System in the dying process. Emphasis should be on clear elucidation of the Hope System of (1) the nurse-practitioner, (2) the dying patient, and (3) the family of the dying person. The second phase should contain methods to clarify and effectively support the patient's Hope System so that his needs will be met in a realistic and holistic manner.

Utilizing the Hope System as a frame of reference as well as responding to the basic needs of the dying person will enable us to more meaningfully interact with patients and assist them to complete their lives in a natural and holistic manner.

Alternate Methods of Treatment

It is most important that a discussion of this nature include some alternate methods of treatment to augment current medical regimens in the care of the dying.

Meditation

Meditation is a mode of assisting the dying person to relax. It facilitates the effects of pain medication and increases the medication's effectiveness and duration. Thus, meditation has proven extremely useful in persons with metastatic bone disease. Also, forms of meditation that enable dying persons to get in touch with their deeper selves and spiritual levels have facilitated the transition into the Hope for a Peaceful Death phase. Thus, persons in the final stage of the life continuum are assisted by using meditation to separate from family and significant others with less trauma than persons not utilizing this approach.

Biofeedback

Biofeedback techniques have also been useful in assisting patients undergoing a variety of current treatment modalities, such as radiation therapy and several chemotherapy protocols, to control or prevent the nausea and vomiting that are sometimes associated with these treatment modalities. Becoming aware of all the natural feedback systems of the body has been utilized to assist dying patients to become more aware of the beginnings of pain and has guided them in more effective regulation of pain medication as well as some of the other medications to decrease symptoms.

Visualization

Visualization is a technique utilized by Dr. C. Simonton and others that has been extremely effective in the care of cancer patients, particularly as they near the final stage in the life continuum.[2] Visualization techniques described here have been most effective with patients who have progressive tumor growth that is considered inoperable due to the size and mass of the tumor itself. The patients are instructed to actually visualize the tumor and think of it as being broken up into small pieces from within by power of their own thoughts, being carried away by the bloodstream, and passed out and excreted by the individual. Visualization and imagery of this kind have decreased the tumor mass significantly in some patients so as to allow for surgical intervention.

Utilization of this newer technique with cancer patients undergoing radiation therapy and chemotherapy in conjunction with established medical treatment modalities has produced effects on several levels and in many cases has had a more total and holistic effect on the individual. This is accomplished by instructing the patient to visualize destruction and disintegration of the tumor by cobalt or chemical means as the patient receives the treatment or injection. The method has enabled the person undergoing these treatments to become more of a partner in the therapy rather than a passive recipient in the treatment process. Active inclusion of the patient on the mental level helps create an open mind and a more positive attitude, and acts as a trigger mechanism to bring the patient's own natural immune system into play. The result of this partnership with the patient, plus a multilevel approach, has been to render the treatment modalities more effective in shrinking the tumor with less total dosage and has decreased the length of time the patient must receive chemotherapeutic agents.

Visualization by the nurse, by the patients, and by the family of a white light or blue light that bathes and actually suffuses the patient has been utilized to decrease the terrible anxiety that increases as death approaches, to give comfort to the dying person, and to actually assist the person in the transition we call death. Use of combined therapy and the interaction produced by Therapeutic Touch and visualization of a blue light down the patient's spinal column that follows nerve pathways to the rest of the body has been effective in penetrating the patient on a very deep level, facilitating the transformation where a person can let go of life. As this occurs, the Hope for a Peaceful Death becomes predominant with the patient letting go of life at a very deep level. It is important to think of the heart when visualizing color, since this is where the letting go of life with all its significant relationships occurs.[3]

The healing or making whole of death is accomplished by assisting the patient to let go of life with as little death trauma as possible, just as we are taught to assist the infant into life with as little birth trauma as possible.[4] It is peace and acceptance that decrease the death trauma. Peace for the dying is the absence of pain on all levels; that is, the absence of physical, mental, emotional, and psychological pain.

Clinical Examples

The following are two cases from the department of radiation therapy at the hospital where I was a member of the nursing staff. The purpose of these is to illustrate the use of imagery and visualization with patients using radiotherapy or chemotherapy.

The first patient, Mrs. C., is a patient who had presented with lymphoma and who had been treated with total nodal irradiation. When she presented again it was for a second primary of the tonsillar area. The patient, after receiving the treatment to only the head and neck area, began to experience the same exact symptoms as when she was treated with total nodal therapy (*i.e.*, nausea and vomiting). After explaining the technique and discussing it with her, I asked her to choose an image of good overcoming evil. The image she chose was that of the Blessed Mother with her arms outstretched and beams of light coming from her hands overcoming the evil which the patient visualized in the form of a snake. Mrs. C. began using this image, and I taught her to visualize it prior to the time of the treatment and at night before going to bed in order to have her intensify the cumulative effects of the radiation. After the second day of active visualization prior to treatment and before bedtime, the side-effects of nausea and vomiting completely subsided, never to return. The act of coming to the department for radiotherapy after having been treated there before acted as a trigger with this patient and brought forth all the old memories. The creation of a new image to counteract the old, as well as the symbolism of good overcoming evil, was extremely important to this patient and decreased the side-effects from her treatment.

The most important use of visualization as I see it in cancer patients is that the use of visualization and imagery triggers their own internal immune response, which is very important in so many debilitated and ill patients to help them through their therapy. It is their first step in inner healing.

The second patient, Mr. D., presented with a massive lung lesion. He was treated with radiotherapy and did not respond to the therapy. It was during the time of the nonresponse that I began working with Mr. D. and his wife, utilizing imagery. They had purchased the book *Getting Well Again* by Carl Simonson and were reading it. I asked the patient to do something which is essential for this technique: to choose his own image of good overcoming evil (*i.e.*, health overcoming illness). The image he chose, since he was an avid golfer, was that of a 7 iron. When I questioned him about the 7 iron he said he chose a 7 iron because it gets you out of the rough, it hacks away at the rough, and he transmuted that image into hacking away at the tumor. The second image, which is equally important, was the visualization of a little wheelbarrel coming up and taking away the particles of tumor that the 7 iron had chopped away and carrying the particles out of his body. His wife's image was that of a miner dressed in a miner's hat with a big light searching the lung and using a pick axe to go after the tumor. However, in the wife's image, she also became very angry, and as pieces of the tumor fell, she would grind them into the ground of the lung in order to kill them. Then she visualized a little car on the tracks in the mine coming and picking up the pieces of tumor like pieces of coal and carrying them out.

After about two weeks this patient was again treated with radiotherapy and there was a marvelous change in the response, so much so that the physician was amazed. Two weeks after beginning, Mr. D. said to me "You know, Cathy, I've been doing what you said, but I want to change the image." He changed the image from a 7 iron to a garden instrument that is V-shaped and goes down deep into the ground and kills the root of dandelions. Then he visualized the dandelions (*i.e.*, tumors) being pulled out of the ground and put in the wheelbarrel. He said he changed the image because there was too much pleasure attached to the use of the 7 iron and he felt he needed something that would get more at the root of his tumor and his problem. Also, after discussing with the patient's wife the possible negative effect of the anger in grinding the tumor into the lung bed and keeping it in the patient, I discussed the anger component with her and she changed her image. In her new image she took the tumor out of the lung and visualized the little pieces of tumor as balloons; she imagined that she released the balloons by cutting the strings to let them go, and they floated out and were taken out of the patient as he breathed in and out. Thus the disease process would then be breathed out of him.

I used the time of treatment as a focal point. I had not only the husband and wife think of wholeness and wellness, but I also contacted their son in Arizona and another son in California. At the same time as the treatment here in New York they also thought of wholeness and wellness to this patient. The response was technically remarkable. There was a decrease in the tumor size and density and also in the size of the nodules. The metastatic nodules to the periphery of the right lung also disappeared.

I also utilized color with this patient because I felt that it was a very significant image. I asked him to find something of a color blue that had vibrance as well as a calming effect on him, since when his tumor at first did not respond to the radiotherapy he needed something else to calm him. A friend of his gave him a little blue duck and that is what he used to visualize color. He put it on his dresser to think of before going to bed at night, and visualizing the image of the blue going through him and permeating him seemed to help him sleep.

To me the most crucial thing in utilizing visualization is that the patient must choose his own image. The image must have significance and symbolization. The emotion of anger has to be dealt with in some way and let go of in order to trigger even more effectively the patient's immune response if there is too heavy an emotional component that can interfere with healing.

Involvement of the family at this very crucial time is important. Instead of being a traumatic, fearful, alien experience, whether it is radiotherapy, as I have described, or chemotherapy, the more the patient and family can form an alliance with the cobalt or the drug treatment, the more effectively they can integrate these toxic things into their own immune systems and use them as an adjunct to healing.

The third patient, whom I will discuss briefly, was a young man with T-cell lymphoblastic lymphoma. He was a very visual young man, and he visualized the tumors in the lymph system as groups of interlocking T's all joined together, some smaller and some larger. He visualized the chemotherapy and also the radiotherapy as being like a hand grenade thrown into this mesh of T's. The mesh of T's would be exploded and blown up, and then the white blood cells would come as what he called the "blue army" and they would take the T's out of him. This young man responded quite well to chemotherapy and radiotherapy; however, the nature of his disease was such that it changed from being predominantly lymphoma to being leukemia. The most interesting change in this patient was that when confronted and given the support of people who cared about him, even when confronted with the terrible blow of leukemia, he changed from a negative self-depreciating young man into a man who wanted to live and grow and wanted to die as a man. It was his own feeling that his negative attitude had planted the seed, had prepared the ground for the seed of the disease to grow and develop, and that actually in some way he had given himself cancer. The use of the image of breaking the cells open and breaking the interlocking lymphoma T that held him in bondage was very significant in freeing his inner person to come to new knowledge and development, and to die free.

Autosuggestion

In autosuggestion, patients are assisted by means of hypnosis, medications, or simply the human voice to go back and visualize themselves as they were before they became ill. For example, a woman who now has a tumor of the breast is assisted by the human voice or by hypnosis to go back in time to her own development as a woman, imagining herself first as a young woman, then as she has continued to age, picturing herself as whole and complete and balanced with both breasts the same as they were before the discovery of the lump. This method has been effective in assisting people to solidify their own mental image and maintain their own self-image despite disfiguring surgery that has altered their physical appearance.

Music Therapy

A modality that has been useful, especially with patients who have extreme pain, is music therapy. Many studies have been done on the actual rhythms in certain musical selections and their effect on the person.[5] It appears that there are certain wave lengths in nature and in sound that are exactly the same as the wave lengths in the muscles. We know that the beginning of pain causes a tightening of the musculature followed by compression of the nerves, which aggravates the pain. On the physiologic level, use of music therapy to relax the muscles has enabled patients to divert or prevent the pain from taking hold of them by preventing compression of nerve roots. This therapy has proved very useful in patients who have a liking for music and who when questioned state that music has always had a calming and relaxing effect on them. It is important to the patient to bring in past experiences and correlate these experiences with what they are experiencing now. Secondly, music with different tempos acts as a distraction, assisting patients to divert their conscious attention from what is really causing the pain. Enlisting the patient's assistance in the choice of familiar or favorite melodies helps the patient assume more responsibility for the treatment process and its effect.

Therapeutic Touch

Touch is not the sole province of nursing. It is a subtle, though universal, signal among humans for expression of empathy, of compassion, of friendliness. We have all had this experience, if from no other persons than certainly from our mothers and fathers or those significantly close to us at some stage in our becoming, such as our friends, our guides, or others. Anybody who has undergone any experiences of self, ranging from structured self-analysis to the fantasies of creative imagery, knows how important the touch of another can be.[6]

The fact that touch is one of the earliest sensations perceived in the birth process clearly demonstrates the importance of this stimulation in the beginning of the life continuum. Actually, touch appears to be essential in freeing the infant from the confines of the womb and assisting him in the birth process that signals the transition into life. Needless to say, there is a whole evolution of touch experiences from hand–mouth exploration to hand–eye coordination that are built into the very fiber of human growth and development during the chronological wave of the ensuing life process. Human touch remains significant throughout our entire lives; indeeed, it is impossible to imagine how we could live without it. Because touch is such an integral part of the entire life process begun at birth, let us now turn our attention to a very important mode of touch as a therapeutic modality that has great significance at the end of the life process, which we call death.

Therapeutic Touch, also known as the laying on of hands, is an actual energy exchange by which the healer, the nurse–healer in this case, actually transduces energy through self to the patient and stimulates the patient's own healing potential.[7] This may be employed for a variety of problems. Therapeutic Touch has proven extremely effective when performed by the nurse as an additive or alternative to traditional therapeutics with dying patients who are having pain, who have edematous extremities, or who are extremely anxious.

The following excerpt from my journal demonstrates the integration of Therapeutic Touch into our modern-day health-care system. It was written when I was a clinical nursing specialist with rehabilitation patients and persons nearing the end of their lives. The journal traces the decrease of bilateral 4-plus edema to no edema over a 4-day period in a patient with metastatic bone disease. The decrease was monitored by measuring the patient's legs, ankles, and knees twice a day. It is important to note that the patient had no cardiovascular impairment and was not on diuretics of any kind.

> The following is a remarkable occurrence with a patient of mine. Mr. A. had primary cancer of the prostate and now presented with metastatic disease of the bone. His legs were very edematous (bilateral 4-plus pitting edema) and I was teaching him quadriceps-setting exercises and passive range-of-motion exercises as part of a maintenance program following a spinal fusion because of lytic lesions.
>
> As I exercised him, I consciously integrated the principles of Therapeutic Touch, thinking of flow throughout the body as a whole, and of a return to wholeness and balance within the patient. I also taught the patient's wife and the nursing staff the technique and its importance. The patient's wife was able to do Therapeutic Touch with her husband several times in the evening. This increased her participation in his care and comfort. The edema was remarkably decreased and one of the nurses said, "Oh, that was because he was on Lasix." His primary nurse said, "But he wasn't on Lasix." I didn't need to say a word since they knew what I was doing.

Now, just a few words about methods of explaining Therapeutic Touch to the clients and the nature of their involvement in this aspect of their total care. It is very important that the nurse–practitioners establish a contract with their clients, explaining to them what they are doing and why they think it will help. To enlist a patient's participation as well as to trigger the patient's own internal healing potential, the nurse must have the patient think of flow and wholeness while the nurse actually does Therapeutic Touch and then intermittently during the day to retain the effect of the energy transfer and stimulate the patient's own healing. This approach truly incorporates patients in their own care and comfort and returns a measure of control over their own bodies to patients who have had much of this self-control taken from them by the disease as well as by the health-care system.

Remember that this cannot be done without the patients permission because that would be a violation of their dignity. One of the phrases that has been helpful to me in introducing Therapeutic Touch to patients is the following: "I have learned something in my nursing education that has been effective with other patients and I think it might help you. It is a very soothing and gentle technique. I will incorporate it with your care and exercises to help you heal and return to health." Inclusion of the patients and their families in this manner seems to help them regain some of their self-esteem and dignity, as well as the control mentioned earlier.

It is important for the nurse–practitioners to note in their journals their patients' subjective responses to the treatment as well as the objective data obtained (*e.g.,* measuring a patient's extremities twice daily and listing all medications, *etc.*). Clients' responses are oftentimes the most interesting and affirming. Mr. A. used to say to me, "You know, it's different when you touch my legs and work with them, it feels different than when anyone else touches them. I feel them getting lighter and they seem more alive to me."

We know that many patients in the last stages of the life process exhibit symptoms or signs of depression and withdrawal as they begin to take their final inner journey preparatory to death. At this time, owing to the great mental and physical pain that patients are experiencing, it is sometimes not possible to actually touch the patients. The nurse–healers using Therapeutic Touch do not need to make contact with the patients in order to be effective. Merely by the nurse's moving his or her hands over a patient's body in a motion that follows the normal blood flow, lymph drainage systems, and neural pathways stimulating normal function has proven effective in decreasing pain and edema, thereby increasing the comfort of the patient. The interaction of the patient and nurse expressed by Therapeutic Touch is the external symbol of the establishment of a trusting relationship wherein the patient knows there is freeing and support at the same time. The nurse–patient interaction becomes extremely significant at this time since many other members of the health-care team may have abandoned the patient.

Megavitamin Therapy

An adjunct therapy that should be utilized more often with cancer patients and with dying persons is megavitamin therapy. Since advanced cancer patients are so depleted on many levels owing to the aggressive nature of the treatment modalities (*i.e.,* radiation therapy, chemotherapy, cortisone, and hormone therapy), this particular group of patients will benefit even more than normal persons from high vitamin intake. Many dying patients with metastatic disease have continual nerve pain and the B vitamins are effective in lessening this pain.

The Hospice

The hospice is a concept that originated in England with Dr. Cecily Saunders and finally is gaining importance here in the United States. Hospices are places where terminally ill patients come not to die but to live each day until they die. The structure of the hospice is very comfortable, and the institution is more like a home than a hospital. Nevertheless, the total care aspect is apparent because the personnel working there provide a compassionate professional background and support system.

The prime need of advanced cancer patients and dying persons is pain control. The pharmacist, physicians, and nurses on the team make this their first priority, for it is impossible for anyone to interact or talk in a therapeutic manner with a patient who has extreme pain. It is essential that the pain be controlled in order to enable the patient to relate to you on other levels. Clergymen also form part of the team because so many of the needs of dying persons have to do with religion and with finishing their business.

The philosophy of care for any hospice concept, whether it be a free-standing edifice inpatient unit or a hospice home care approach, must possess the following as elements of care*:

It is our primary responsibility to respond to, and assure that the needs of the advanced cancer patient are attended to. The first and most basic need is that the terminally ill patient needs to

*Fanslow C: Philosophy of Nursing Care. Adopted by the Council on Nursing Practice, May 4, 1979; approved by the New York State Nursing Association, June 21, 1979. Albany, New York State Nurses Association, 1979. Used with permission.

know he will not be abandoned. The contract between patient, family and care-giver is solidified by the establishing and maintenance of the trusting relationship, wherein the patient is assured that he will not be abandoned on any level, at any time.

He and his family know that he will be cared for physically with respect, gentleness of touch and dignity of approach. He will be cared for psychologically by the presence of staff who are able and willing to listen to his cries for help and support, enabling him to finish his business, say his goodbyes and the necessary "I love you" that will free him to leave, and spiritually, by the healing words, blessings and communion which bring with it a "peace no man can give and strength for the final journey."

He will be cared for humanely by being able to touch, share and create life, by participating in play and re-creation until he is ready and able to let go of it, and by insuring that he exercise as much control over his life, body, play and dreams as he wishes to, until he graciously and freely allows us to assist him in his task.

• • •

His death must be peaceful, meaning that he die, no, not only die, but live as free from pain each day until he dies. The absence of pain must be, first and foremost, freedom from physical pain; second, freedom from the psychological pain of isolation and abandonment; third, freedom from the spiritual pain of alienation; lastly, freedom from the human pain of loss of vitality and control which makes one dependent and unable to participate in life.

Our philosophy of care must create and allow the external environment and contain the internal trust relationship wherein the fundamental needs of the dying person are respected, listened to, protected and assured so that our patients will be assisted to truly and freely live each day until they die.[8]

It would be proper for us as a profession to foster the hospice concept and, if possible, become instrumental in establishing hospices here in the United States. Let us go back to our historical perspectives when patients were nursed and cared for and then died in the very homes that they had been born in. Ideally a hospice most nearly approximates the home environment while providing the necessary support systems which at times the normal family of today does not possess. That is, support family members who are not sufficiently prepared to deal with the patient's pain, whether it be physical, mental, psychological, emotional, or spiritual. Most often families find it impossible to give the necessary support to the dying person. Because of their involvement with the dying person and the fact that this person is leaving them, they themselves are in pain.

Summary

What I have attempted to do in this chapter is assist beginning nurse-practitioners in taking an inward journey consisting of confrontation and exploration of their own personal experiences with death and their effect on them as humans. I have tried to outline methods that will help beginning practitioners grow and develop into effective instruments in the care of the dying.

It is essential that all those who will have the singular privilege of caring for the dying be taught to take this significant inward journey in order to assist people to die as well as they can and to ensure that their basic needs, the need for nonabandonment and the need for hope, are sustained.

All approaches and intervention are supportive of the basic fact that death is a part of life, part of the wellness spectrum. Indeed, one might say that death is the completion of life itself and should be treated with as much, or more, respect as the beginning of life.

Training Methods in Awareness

A variety of methods may be used to assist nurses in becoming aware of their own attitudes, feelings, and fears toward the dying and death.

I have found a questionnaire to be a controllable and effective method of assisting health-care professionals to focus their feelings and responses on the dying process. The value of this method is that, being able to respond by written answers to questions, students examine their feelings and fears more objectively than they might be able to in direct verbal communication and in other teaching situations. After the students have given thought to their responses and placed them on paper, an in-depth discussion follows with verbalization of responses. In addition, on the basis of student responses, the leader can redirect discussion and encourage greater exploration and verbalization of feelings.

The sample questions that I have found especially helpful on questionnaires are listed in the Experiential Exercises.

The activities described in the Experiential Exercises also are useful in helping individuals develop a holistic perspective toward dying and death as parts of the life continuum. Other effective exercises are role-playing and case studies. They increase nurses' awareness of their interactions and intervention with terminally ill patients and their families.

Post-death conferences initiated shortly after a patient has died offer an opportunity for the staff and students to examine their feelings and approach to patient and family. These conferences minimize emotional buildup, internalization of feelings of failure, and negative feelings toward one's self. It is most helpful for the instructor or for the students themselves to select practical situations on the patient unit which provide an opportunity to apply knowledge acquired during role-play and case-study sessions.

The utilization of audiovisual presentations in the absence of patient accessibility has also proved an effective method to prepare beginning health-care practitioners. There are many audiovisual aids available. Concept Media film strip presentations are one of the most realistic and effective audiovisual aids that can be used to assist students in this area

All the methods described here have been included for the primary purpose of assisting beginning student nurses to explore their feelings toward death so that they may intervene appropriately with terminally ill patients and their families. A secondary purpose is to provide the beginning practitioner with an understanding and awareness of the dying process as a part of the total holistic perspective of man.

Experiential Exercises

Sample Questions for Questionnaires

1. Death became a reality to me at the age of _____ when _____ died.
   (person, animal)

2. I felt _____ (about this death)

3. If today I were told I have a fatal illness, I would probably _____ .

4. I (would/would not) want my family to know that I have a fatal illness because _____ .

5. If I need help in facing death, the person I would trust most would be _____ .

6. I have the most trouble talking to a dying person when

   _____ .

7. I wish there was some way I could help families to _____ .

Activities

1. Make a list of whom you would want to come to your funeral and why you would like them there.

2. State what you want to be remembered for and by whom.

3. List in order those people who would miss you and why.
4. Formulate a list of those whom you would miss the most and why.
5. Describe your death (when, why, how, and where).
6. Discuss your death preference as to time: quick, slow; no time to prepare; some time to prepare; long time to prepare.
7. Write in detail your last will and testament.
8. Write your own obituary for the local newspaper.

References

1. Kübler-Ross E: On Death and Dying. New York, Macmillan, 1969
2. Simonton C: Use of meditation and visualization in the care of terminal cancer patients. Cancer Res 76:478–86, 1976
3. Steiner R: Colour. London, Rudolf Steiner Press, 1971
4. Meek GW: Healers and the Healing Process. A Quest Book. Wheaton, Ill, Theosophical Publishing House, 1977
5. Bonny H, Savary L: Music and Your Mind: Listening With a New Consciousness. New York, Harper & Row, 1973
6. Krieger D: Therapeutic touch: the imprimatur of nursing. Am Nurs 75:784–787, 1975
7. Krieger D: The Therapeutic Touch: How to Use Your Hands to Help or to Heal. Englewood Cliffs, Prentice-Hall, 1979
8. Fanslow CA: Care of the Dying. Written in Collaboration with the New York State Nurses Associateion Council on Nursing Practice. Albany, New York State Nurses Association, 1979

Suggested Readings

Blue A, Savary L: Horizons of Hope, the Quest for a New Consciousness. Minnesota, St. Mary's College Press, 1969
Browning MH, Lewis EP: The Dying Patient: a Nursing Perspective. New York, the American Journal of Nursing Company, 1972
Carroll J: Elements of Hope. New Jersey, Paulist Press, 1972
Caughill RE (ed): The Dying Patient: a Supportive Approach. Boston, Little, Brown, 1976
Chaney PS: Dealing With Death and Dying. Nursing '77, Skillbook Series. Horsham, Pa, Intermed Communications, 1977
Dempsey D: The Way We Die. New York, McGraw-Hill, 1975
Earle AM, Argandizzo NT, Kutscher A: In Kutscher AH (ed): The Nurse as Caregiver for the Terminal Patient and His Family. New York, Columbia University Press, 1976
Feifel H (ed): The Meaning of Death. New York, McGraw-Hill, 1969
Hinton J: Dying. New York, Penguin Books, 1974
Kastenbaum R: Death, Society, and Human Experience. St Louis, CV Mosby, 1977

Kastenbaum R, Aisenberg R: The Psychology of Death. New York, Springer, 1972

Keleman S: Living Your Dying. New York, Random House, 1975

Krieger D: The Therapeutic Touch. Englewood Cliffs, Prentice-Hall, 1979

Kübler-Ross E: On Death and Dying. New York, Macmillan, 1969

Kübler-Ross E: Death the Final Stage of Growth. Englewood Cliffs, Prentice-Hall, 1975

Simonton C, et al: Getting Well Again. California, JP Tarcher, 1978

Steiner R: Colour. London, Rudolf Steiner, 1971

Strauss B, Glaser R: Awareness of Dying. New York, Macmillan, 1971

Teirich HR: Therapeutics Through Music and Vibration. H Scherschen,

Villaverde MM, Wright C, : Pain From Symptom to Treatment. Litton Educational Publishing, 1977

Weisman AD: On Dying and Denying. New York, Behavioral Publications, 1972

Index

Page numbers followed by t refer to tables.